- Do you overeat?
- Are you unable to sleep at night?
- Do you feel anxious and fearful for no apparent reason?
- Are you often moody or depressed?
- Do you find that you're forgetful or unable to concentrate?
- Does the idea of using prescription drugs concern you?

IF YOU ANSWERED "YES" TO ANY OF THESE QUESTIONS, LEARN THE **SECRETS OF 5-HTP** AND FIND OUT IF THIS AMAZING NATURAL SUPPLEMENT IS RIGHT FOR YOU!

SECRETS OF
5-HTP

WINIFRED CONKLING

A LYNN SONBERG BOOK

St. Martin's Paperbacks

The twelve steps of the Overeaters Anonymous program on pp. 82–84 are reprinted by permission of Overeaters Anonymous, Inc.
Copyright © 1980 by Overeaters Anonymous, Inc.
All rights reserved.

SECRETS OF 5-HTP

ISBN: 0-312-96859-0

Printed in the United States of America

St. Martin's Paperbacks edition / November 1998

St. Martin's Paperbacks are published by St. Martin's Press, 175 Fifth Avenue, New York, NY 10010.

10 9 8 7 6 5 4 3 2 1

AUTHOR'S NOTE

CONTENTS

CONTENTS

PART III: USING 5-HTP

INTRODUCTION

THIS BOOK WILL LET YOU IN ON THE SECRETS OF 5-HTP, a simple nutritional supplement that can have a profound influence on your mood, your eating habits, your sleep patterns, and your overall health. In fact, its impressive performance in treating a wide range of health problems has made it one of the hottest new supplements available in health food stores today.

5-HTP works by creating subtle but significant changes in your brain's chemistry. Specifically, it increases the levels of the neurotransmitter serotonin in the brain. It would be difficult to overestimate the importance of serotonin to your physical and mental health. Serotonin is one of the body's most important modulators of mood, appetite, sleep, and impulse control. Low levels of serotonin have been linked to depression, bulimia, anorexia, overeating, insomnia, anxiety, migraine headaches, and seasonal affective disorder, among other health problems.

Because inadequate serotonin levels can trigger a number of different problems, it comes as no surprise that many of these conditions overlap in the same person. For example, depression and alcoholism have been found to run in families, and some researchers have suggested that there may be an inherited problem with serotonin functioning. The same is true for migraine headaches and depression. In addition, a number of studies of people suffering from the eating disorder bulimia nervosa have found that they have a higher-than-average frequency of mood disorders (depression or anxiety) and substance abuse problems. In many cases physicians and therapists find it difficult or impossible to determine the primary or root cause of a patient's problems when he or she suffers from a number of different problems.

To treat people with these problems, medical doctors often prescribe drugs designed to tinker with brain chemistry by raising serotonin levels. Each year, millions of Americans boost their serotonin levels by taking drugs known as selective serotonin reuptake inhibitors (SSRIs), such as Prozac (fluoxetine), Zoloft (sertraline), and Paxil (paroxetine). Other drugs that use a similar mechanism include the antianxiety drug Buspar (buspirone) and the antimigraine medication Imitrex (sumatriptan). Because these drugs help to raise serotonin levels as a means of treating one condition, they often prove useful at treating other, seemingly unrelated conditions. For example, drugs used to treat depression are often successful at preventing migraines, or stopping binge eating, because all of these conditions can be caused by low levels of serotonin in the brain.

Although prescription drugs may be necessary for the treatment of some patients, they usually are expensive and all have side effects. In many cases, people can raise their serotonin levels naturally, without turning to prescription drugs. The secret, of course, is 5-HTP!

5-HTP (5-hydroxy L-tryptophan) is the link between the foods we eat and serotonin in the brain. It is produced by the body from the amino acid tryptophan, which is found in many of the foods we eat, such as dairy products and meat. In the body, 5-HTP is then broken down into the neurotransmitter serotonin. By taking 5-HTP as a nutrition supplement, you provide your body with the materials it needs to convert this simple substance into health-enhancing serotonin in the brain.

This book explains how 5-HTP works in the body—and how it can work for you. Part I, "Understanding 5-HTP," explains how the tryptophan, 5-HTP, and serotonin work together to affect brain chemistry and behavior. Part II, "Consider the Evidence," outlines the relationship between serotonin levels and a number of medical problems and presents the research on how 5-HTP has been used to boost serotonin and promote healing. Finally, Part III, "Using 5-HTP," provides details on the safe and effective use of 5-HTP for a variety of health problems.

Of course, the information presented here is not intended to take the place of consultation with a trained medical professional. Always consult your doctor before using 5-HTP to improve your condition, especially if you suffer from severe depression, eating disorders, anxiety, or insomnia. (A list of resources for more information on various medical problems is included in each section.)

Part 1

UNDERSTANDING 5-HTP

1. KEEPING THE BALANCE: 5-HTP, SEROTONIN, AND BRAIN CHEMISTRY

To APPRECIATE THE MIRACLE OF 5-HTP, YOU must first appreciate the miracle that is your brain. Once you have a basic understanding of the way the brain works, you will be better able to understand how the nutrition supplement 5-HTP can have such a profound effect on mood and behavior.

The pathways of communication in the brain are almost unimaginably complex. The numbers can be difficult to grasp, but researchers estimate that between 10 and 100 billion neurons exist in the human brain, and each of those neurons connects to thousands of others. Amazingly, this intricate communication network operates without any direct connections—all those neurons pass their messages from one to another without touching. Instead, they rely on neurotransmitters, biochemicals designed to act like chemical postal workers, passing messages between neurons with remarkable speed and accuracy.

Between each of the neurons is a microscopic space known as the synaptic gap. In order to communicate, the neuron releases a tiny burst of electric current, which zips through the neuron and releases a cluster of chemical neurotransmitter molecules stored at the base of the neuron in tiny sacs known as vesicles. After they have been freed, the neurotransmitters make their way across the synaptic gap and work their way into the receptor sites of the neighboring neuron. Not every neurotransmitter "fits" with every neuron; a particular neurotransmitter can activate only those receptor types designed to receive it.

Once a sufficient number of neurotransmit-

ters have been passed on to the receiving neuron, this neuron sends out its own electric
charge, and the process repeats itself as part
of a biochemical relay race. After sending
their message, the neurotransmitters detach
and return to the original neuron to be reabsorbed.

When the neurotransmitters are in good
supply, the system works well. However, if
there is a shortage of the necessary neurotransmitters, the system breaks down and
neurological messages go undelivered. As a
result, some brain circuits are underactivated,
while others are overactivated.

THE IMPORTANCE OF SEROTONIN

Serotonin is one of most important of the ten
major neurotransmitters in the brain. All of
the neurotransmitters work together to help
us make decisions, formulate our thoughts,
and clarify our perceptions. Many different
parts of the brain participate in making important decisions, such as when we eat and
sleep, how we feel, how much energy we

have, and whether we are motivated to take action on a given matter. The decision-making process would break down into chaos if serotonin didn't help to control and modulate the effect of the other neurotransmitters. In the words of Northwestern University psychiatrist James Stockard, "A person's mood is like a symphony, and serotonin is like the conductor's baton."

Serotonin is a very powerful neurotransmitter, which is known to be able to "unlock" or "fit into" at least fourteen different receptor sites. These receptor sites directly control human mood and behavior. The fact that serotonin fits so many different receptor sites may help to explain why this neurotransmitter is able to influence so much of the human psyche and so many different behaviors, from depression to eating disorders to migraine headaches.

When it comes to the effect of serotonin on mood, researchers have found that the neurotransmitter helps to promote feelings of well-being, calm, personal security, relaxation, confidence, and concentration. In addition, serotonin helps offset the impact of two other neurotransmitters (dopamine and norepinephrine), which can cause feelings of anxiety, fear, anger, tension, aggression, violence, obsessive-compulsive actions, overeating, and sleep disturbances.

When you appreciate the important role that serotonin plays in the brain, then it comes as no surprise that people with low levels of serotonin in the brain often suffer from a range of problems, including depression, anxiety, insomnia, violence, eating disorders, migraine headaches, premenstrual syndrome, seasonal affective disorder, compulsive behaviors (such as compulsive gambling and compulsive sex), and alcoholism, among others. In many cases, relief from these mental, emotional, and behavioral problems can be achieved by increasing levels of serotonin in the brain.

PRESCRIPTION DRUGS AND
SEROTONIN LEVELS

This book discusses ways you can use the nutritional supplement 5-HTP to raise serotonin levels. Even though this natural approach is highly effective, millions of Americans instead choose to boost their serotonin levels through the use of prescription drugs.

Drugs that boost serotonin levels enter the brain and mimic the serotonin molecule by tricking the receptor on the neighboring neurotransmitter into responding. Other drugs work by blocking the receptor and preventing it from receiving incoming messages from other molecules. Still other drugs work by blocking the production of the neurotransmitters themselves.

The popular class of drugs known as selective serotonin reuptake inhibitors includes Prozac, Zoloft, and Paxil. These drugs work by allowing serotonin to be recycled by the body. Under typical circumstances, after serotonin delivers its message it is reabsorbed or taken up by the neuron that released it. SSRIs work their magic by interfering with the reabsorption (reuptake) of the serotonin, leaving more serotonin in circulation so that it is available to deliver its message more than once. In this way, SSRIs increase serotonin activity without necessarily increasing serotonin production in the brain.

The success of SSRIs hinges on the ability of the body to produce an adequate amount of serotonin in the brain. 5-HTP, on the other hand, naturally elevates the levels of serotonin in the brain, increasing serotonin activity without the side effects associated with the use of SSRIs.

THE SIDE EFFECTS OF SSRIS

On the whole, SSRIs tend to have fewer side effects than many other drugs used to treat depression and serotonin-dependent conditions, but these drugs still have many more side effects than 5-HTP.

Consider this list of possible side effects for Prozac and the other SSRIs:

- *Prozac can encourage suicide attempts in depressed people first taking the drug.* Prozac may facilitate suicidal behavior in a small number of people who considered suicide but were too depressed to act on their feelings. After taking Prozac for a couple of weeks, these people felt energized enough to act on their negative emotions, but they had not been on the drug long enough to enjoy its mood-enhancing benefits. Doctors now realize that there may be a "window of vulnerability" two to six weeks after a person begins taking SSRIs during which he or she may be vulnerable to acting on suicidal feelings.

- *About half of the men and women taking Prozac and other SSRIs experience problems with sexual function*, most often decrease in libido (or sexual desire) and delayed orgasm. The problems for men include failure to ejaculate, painful ejaculation, and impotence.

- *Prozac can cause agitation.* Clinical trials indicate that about 15 percent of people taking Prozac experience nervousness, and another 10 percent experience anxiety. In most cases, lowering the dose of the drug doesn't ease these symptoms.

- *SSRIs can cause insomnia and sleep disturbances.* About 15 percent of people taking Prozac experience insomnia in the early weeks of treatment. The other SSRIs tend to cause similar problems, with one exception, the SSRI known as Serzone.

- *SSRIs can cause drowsiness.* While some people experience agitation, others become drowsy. About one out of every five people taking SSRIs feels sleepy during the day.

- *SSRIs can cause tension and migraine headaches.* About 20 percent of the people who take Prozac experience headaches.

- *Prozac can create digestive system problems.* It can cause nausea (21 percent of people on Prozac), diarrhea (12 percent), dry mouth (10 percent), indigestion (6 percent), abdominal pain (3 percent), and vomiting (2 percent).

Again, Prozac and other SSRIs definitely have fewer side effects than the earlier classes of antidepressants, but they can cause a range of annoying symptoms. In contrast, the most common side effect of 5-HTP is gastrointestinal illness. (For more information on side effects of 5-HTP, see Chapter 6, "The Safe and Effective Use of 5-HTP.")

FUELING YOUR BRAIN:
PRODUCING SEROTONIN

If someone is deficient in serotonin, you may wonder, why not just take supplemental serotonin? This reasonable-sounding approach won't work because serotonin cannot pass from the bloodstream into the brain. Instead, serotonin and other neurotransmitters must be produced inside the brain from precursor chemicals or raw ingredients found in foods or nutritional supplements.

This may seem like a cumbersome system, but it protects the brain from toxins and accidental poisonings. The blood-brain barrier isn't a blockade; it prevents some large molecules from crossing into the brain and it slows the progress of others. Serotonin molecules are too big to cross the blood-brain barrier; its precursor, tryptophan, can slip across, but it must wait its turn among the other amino acids also trying to enter the brain. The blood-brain barrier allows amino acids to cross into the brain, but it lets in only a few at a time.

Once they have completed the journey into the brain, amino acids are used by the body to produce specific neurotransmitters. Serotonin (also called 5-HT) is made from tryptophan, an amino acid found in bananas, meat, fish, poultry, nuts, soybeans, brewer's yeast, peanut butter, cooked dried beans, and dairy products. In addition to producing serotonin in the brain, the body uses tryptophan in the blood platelets, the liver, the kidneys, and some cell linings. This serotonin found throughout the body does nothing to alter mood or behavior, because it cannot cross into the brain. For serotonin to affect brain chemistry, it must be produced inside the neurons in the brain.

To produce serotonin, the body needs plenty of tryptophan, but tryptophan is the least plentiful of the twenty-three amino acids found in foods. In most cases, there are seven to nine molecules of other amino acids for every molecule of tryptophan fighting for a place in line to cross the blood-brain barrier into the brain.

You might think that you could increase the levels of tryptophan waiting to cross the blood-brain barrier by eating foods high in tryptophan, but this approach won't work. Tryptophan is often plentiful in high-protein foods, which are packed with a number of other amino acids as well. If you eat these high-protein foods, you actually consume a number of different amino acids, which makes the competition even worse!

Ironically, the secret to increasing tryptophan is to avoid protein and instead eat high-carbohydrate foods. In the body, the carbohydrates cause the pancreas to release insulin to lower the blood sugar levels. This insulin also clears away most of the amino acids waiting in line with tryptophan to cross into the brain. (For more information on diet and tryptophan, see Chapter 7, "Eat Smart: The 5-HTP–Enhancing Diet.")

Millions of Americans practice this eating strategy without appreciating the science behind it. When they feel stressed or depressed, they reach for candy, cake, chips, ice cream, and other high-carbohydrate snack foods. These foods actually do create a passing feeling of well-being and security because they increase levels of serotonin in the brain. Of course, the approach won't work on an ongoing basis because it results in obesity and its related health problems. But it does explain why many people "self-medicate" by using food to adjust their mood.

THE ROLE OF NUTRITIONAL SUPPLEMENTS

Although you cannot take serotonin supplements, you can take other nutritional supplements that are used by the body to create serotonin. In the 1970s and 1980s, millions of Americans took tryptophan supplements to help them sleep, improve their mood, ease

A WORD ABOUT AMINO ACIDS

Tryptophan and 5-HTP are amino acids, the "building blocks of protein." You may remember learning about amino acids in high school biology. Here is a short primer on the role and function of amino acids in the body.

- When amino acids join together in chains, they form proteins. Twenty-two different amino acids have been identified in the human body, and are known to form at least 100,000 different types of proteins in nature.

- The human body consists of more than 50,000 different forms of protein. Amino acids account for three-quarters of the body's dry weight (excluding water).

- Amino acids consist of combinations of carbon, hydrogen, oxygen, nitrogen, and sometimes sulfur.

- Every amino acid comes in two forms, a left-handed (or L-) form and a right-handed (or D-) form. L- and D- amino acids are chemically identical, except that they are the mirror image of each other (just as your left and right hands are mirror images of each other). The human body is constructed of L-amino acids; this book involves the use of L-5-HTP (though we often refer to it simply as 5-HTP since the D-form is not commercially available).

- L-tryptophan is considered an essential amino acid because the body cannot manufacture its own.

- The proteins in foods we eat are broken down into their amino acids in the digestive tract; some of these are then used when proteins are reassembled in the liver.

---

the intensity of obsessions and compulsions, and make other adjustments in mood and behavior attributed to changes in serotonin levels. In the body, supplemental tryptophan is converted into 5-HTP and then into 5-HT, or serotonin.

Not all the tryptophan you ingest (either as food or as nutritional supplements) enters the brain as 5-HTP. Tryptophan can take one of several pathways through the body. Researchers believe that only about 1 percent of the tryptophan taken as a nutritional supplement makes its way across the blood-brain barrier, where it is available for conversion into serotonin in the brain. The remaining 99 percent of the tryptophan is processed in one of several ways. It can be used by the body to make proteins and vitamin B_3, it can be converted into serotonin outside the brain (where it can be used by other cells in the body), or it can be broken down through bodily processes. (An estimated 98 percent of tryptophan is degraded and excreted through the urine.)

Our knowledge of how tryptophan works in the body was steadily growing until the use of tryptophan in the United States came to an abrupt halt in 1989 when the U.S. Food and Drug Administration banned its sale due to a possible health risk. (For more information, see Chapter 2: "The Truth About Tryptophan and 5-HTP.")

Fortunately, a safe, natural, and effective alternative to tryptophan is now known: 5-HTP. As a supplement, 5-HTP is superior to tryptophan for a number of reasons: It is not incorporated into proteins or used to make vitamin B_3 (so more of it is available to increase levels of serotonin in the brain), and, most important, it easily crosses the blood-brain barrier. In other words, 5-HTP is directly and efficiently converted into serotonin in the brain, whereas the majority of tryptophan taken as a supplement is diverted into side missions not related to boosting serotonin levels.

Because 5-HTP is much more efficient than tryptophan, less of it is needed to achieve therapeutic benefits. For example, many studies have found that 100 or 200 milligrams of 5-HTP per day is as effective as 1,000 or 2,000 milligrams of tryptophan.

TOO MUCH OF A GOOD THING

If something is good, more isn't necessarily better. While low levels of serotonin can trigger mood disorders, eating disorders, insomnia, migraines, and other problems, too much serotonin can cause complications as well.

It is possible to overdose on serotonin-active drugs, creating an emergency condition known as "serotonin syndrome." The condition can be difficult to diagnose, but the symptoms include confusion, agitation, profuse sweating, high fever, high blood pressure, and muscle rigidity. Treatment involves

CAN 5-HTP BE MADE MORE EFFECTIVE?

For 5-HTP to boost serotonin in the brain, it must first be able to reach the brain. For a time, researchers worried about the ability of the enzyme L-aromatic amino acid decarboxylase (L-ADD) to convert 5-HTP to serotonin before it enters the brain. (L-ADD is especially active in liver, kidney, and intestinal linings.)

In an attempt to make 5-HTP even more effective, some researchers experimented with the use of compounds called peripheral decarboxylase inhibitors (PDIs) in conjunction with 5-HTP. These PDIs—usually carbidopa or benserazide—prevent the L-ADD from converting 5-HTP to serotonin outside the brain.

The results: 5-HTP is no more effective when used with PDIs, but the PDIs can cause additional side effects. One study treated people with depression using 5-HTP both with and without a PDI. Both treatments proved equally effective, but the group taking the PDI suffered more than twice the number of side effects. The author of the study concluded that "there was no evidence that the administration of benserazide (a PDI) intensified the efficacy of L-5-HTP." A review study of the literature involving experiments using 5-HTP and PDIs found that 5-HTP was actually more effective when given alone in a majority of cases.

administering fluids and medication to control blood pressure. In most cases, the problem passes in a few days, but in several cases it has been fatal.

Most cases of serotonin syndrome involve people who go off a class of antidepressants known as monoamine oxidase (MAO) inhibitors and start taking a different type of antidepressant too soon. (It takes at least two weeks for the MAO inhibitor to clear the system, allowing the person safely to use another type of medication.)

5-HTP will not cause serotonin syndrome, if it is used at the levels described in Chapter 6, "The Safe and Effective Use of 5-HTP." However, if you are taking SSRIs or any other drug that affects serotonin activity, do not use 5-HTP unless your doctor advises you to do so.

2. THE TRUTH ABOUT TRYPTOPHAN AND 5-HTP

TRYPTOPHAN HAS UNFAIRLY EARNED A REPU-tation as a dangerous nutritional supplement. When some consumers learn that the amino acid has been banned by the U.S. Food and Drug Administration, they assume that the product is harmful—and that 5-HTP may be harmful as well, since it is derived from tryptophan. But there is more to the story than this.

For more than twenty years, millions of Americans took tryptophan supplements to treat a number of common health problems, particularly insomnia, depression, and premenstrual syndrome (PMS). At that time, tryptophan enjoyed a positive image as a healthful, natural nutritional supplement that was effective and safer than conventional sleeping pills, antidepressants, or medications for PMS. It was one of the most popular nutritional supplements on the market, and an estimated twelve to thirteen million Americans regularly used tryptophan.

Tryptophan's image was tarnished in 1989 when there was an outbreak of a rare and incurable blood disease among thousands of people taking tryptophan. More than 1,500 people taking the amino acid developed a disease known as eosinophilia-myalgia syndrome (EMS), and at least thirty-eight people died.

EMS derives its name from two distinguishing characteristics of the disease: eosinophilia (because people with the disease have a high number of one kind of white blood cells called eosinophils) and myalgia (because people with EMS suffer from muscle pain). Tragically, more than half of the people who developed EMS after taking the drug have suffered from ongoing painful nerve damage, severe joint pain, fatigue, and scarring of skin and internal organs.

The FDA responded by banning all U.S. sales of tryptophan in early 1990. That ban remains in effect today, although many scientists and informed users of nutritional supplements believe that the ongoing ban is unjustified.

When the tryptophan tragedy was in full swing, researchers from the U.S. Centers for Disease Control and the Mayo Clinic and other leading medical researchers began investigating the crisis. They were able to link many of the problems back to a batch of tryptophan produced by a single Japanese manufacturer. They learned that the company apparently introduced an impurity when it changed its manufacturing process during the first six months of 1989.

The chemical company involved in the crisis was one of six Japanese nutritional supplement manufacturers that produced almost all of the tryptophan used by American consumers. Studies published in 1990 in the *Journal of the American Medical Association* and the *New England Journal of Medicine* pointed fingers at the new recombinant DNA technology used to produce the tryptophan as the most likely source of the problem. Specifically, the articles suggested that a new strain of bacteria might have been responsible for the outbreak of EMS. In other words, leading researchers suspected that the hazards associated with tryptophan stemmed from a contamination problem during the manufacturing process, not from the tryptophan itself.

The FDA remained unconvinced that the entire problem reflected a manufacturing glitch, so it stood behind the ban. It is worth pointing out, however, that while the federal government banned tryptophan as a nutritional supplement, it did not ban its use in other applications. In fact, tryptophan remains an approved ingredient in many infant formulas and intravenous feeding solutions to this day. The U.S. Department of Agriculture allows the use of tryptophan in animal feed, and it can be used in the treatment of animals. In addition, tryptophan is available at a number of U.S. pharmacies, if you can get your doctor to write you a prescription. A nutritional supplement that was safely used by millions of Americans in the 1980s is available only by prescription in the 1990s.

It should also be noted that cases of EMS were rare before 1989, even though millions of Americans regularly used tryptophan. Ironically, some studies even suggest that uncontaminated tryptophan may actually be beneficial in the treatment of EMS.

Many experts consider the tryptophan ban unfair and unnecessary, but it has had one unintended benefit for consumers. It has allowed researchers, manufacturers, and nutritional advocates to focus their attention on 5-HTP, which has not been prohibited by the FDA. And, according to a growing body of literature, 5-HTP is more effective than tryptophan at managing many of the disorders and health problems related to low levels of serotonin in the brain.

If you're interested in boosting your serotonin levels using a natural nutritional supplement (with few unwanted side effects) rather than relying on a prescription drug (with many unwanted side effects), read on. 5-HTP may be the nutritional supplement you've been waiting for—a simple and natural way to improve your mood and your overall health.

Part 2

CONSIDER THE EVIDENCE

3. A NATURAL ALTERNATIVE TO PROZAC: 5-HTP AND DEPRESSION

*With all due deference to scientific skepticism . . .
not to concede 5-HTP its place among acknowl-
edged pharmacotherapeutics routinely applied
against depression does not seem warranted, nei-
ther on empirical nor on theoretical grounds.*

—W. P. Poeldinger, B. Calanchini,
and W. Schwarz, Psychopathology

DEPRESSION AND SADNESS INVOLVE TWO DIFFER-
ent shades of gray. Both involve feelings of
pessimism, apathy, worthlessness, and
gloom. Both involve sensory dullness, in
which food loses its flavor and life loses its
spark of excitement. The difference between
depression and sadness is intensity: Depression is a dark, menacing cloud that blackens
the entire sky and lingers for weeks, while
sadness is a gloomy, overcast day that still al-

lows occasional rays of sunshine to peek through the clouds.

While it can be difficult to distinguish between depression and sadness, both conditions need to be taken seriously—and both tend to respond well to nutritional supplements that boost levels of serotonin in the brain. In fact, depressed moods have been linked to lowered levels of serotonin in the brain. For decades, researchers have demonstrated the connection between mood and serotonin levels, both among people who suffer from severe depression and anxiety and those who experience occasional blue moods or periods of mild depression.

When it comes to monitoring mood, serotonin helps to balance mood shifts and keep us on an even keel. It helps us filter out and ignore unimportant stimulation and to respond appropriately to the issues that should concern us. It helps us avoid depression, anxiety, and suicidal thoughts.

Unfortunately, serotonin does not appear to work as efficiently in women as it does in men. It has been well established that women suffer from depression more often than men, and differences in serotonin synthesis may be the reason. A 1997 study conducted at McGill University in Montreal used positron-emission tomography (PET) to measure rates of serotonin synthesis in the human brain. They found that the mean rate of synthesis in normal (nondepressed) males was 52 percent higher than in normal (nondepressed) females, suggesting that the marked difference may explain the lower incidence of major depression among men.

THE TRYPTOPHAN CONNECTION

Because the body converts tryptophan into 5-HTP and then into serotonin, the amino acid tryptophan can have a powerful influence on our moods. In landmark research done by Dr. George Heninger and Dr. Pedro Delgado, the doctors concocted two different amino acid beverages, one containing all the dietary amino acids found in milk and another containing all of the amino acids except tryptophan. The study participants who drank the beverage containing tryptophan did not experience a dramatic shift in mood, but those who consumed the tryptophan-free drink experienced a 75 percent drop in blood levels of tryptophan—and a dramatic drop in mood. (The people in the study had no history of mood disorders, indicating that the mood shift was a result of the change in tryptophan levels in the body.)

A similar study was performed on people who had been treated for clinical depression in the past but had experienced no current episodes. When those study participants drank the tryptophan-free beverage, fourteen out of twenty-one of them experienced a significant (but short-lived) return of their feelings of depression. One woman in the study had been widowed four years earlier; after drinking the tryptophan-free beverage, she wept and mourned as if she were reexperiencing her husband's death. The next day (after resuming her normal diet), her depression lifted and her mood returned to normal.

Another study published in the British medical journal *The Lancet* in 1997 concluded that people with past episodes of major depression appear to be more vulnerable to tryptophan depletion than people without a history of depression. The mood-lowering effect of tryptophan depletion tends to have a more significant impact on people with a family history of depression, compared to those with a depression-free family tree. Another study conducted at McGill University found that people with no prior episodes of depression but with a multigenerational family history of major affective disorder show a greater reduction in mood after tryptophan depletion.

A population study conducted in 1987 also showed that low tryptophan intakes were linked with increased suicide rates.

Biological studies also support the link between depression and low serotonin levels. In fact, a number of studies have measured markers of serotonin activity in the blood and spinal fluid and found that people suffering from depression also suffer from low serotonin system activity. Suicide has also been associated with decreased serotonin activity.

Although the link between low levels of serotonin and low moods has been firmly established, there is also evidence to suggest that low moods can cause a drop in serotonin system activity. In other words, people can experience depression, only to find the problem made worse because the brain responds by lowering serotonin activity. This hypothesis is supported by researchers who have found that people suffering from post-traumatic stress syndrome and other problems that cause lower serotonin system activity often respond well to treatment with prescription drugs designed to raise serotonin levels.

BOOSTING SEROTONIN—AND MOOD— USING 5-HTP

A number of behavioral and biochemical studies have established a link between 5-HTP and depression.

In fact, a 1991 study published in a Scandinavian psychiatric journal used PET scanning to observe how much 5-HTP reached the brain. As part of the study, eight people with no history of depression and six people diagnosed with major depression were given 5-HTP that had been treated to make it sensitive to the PET-scanning equipment. The researchers found that significantly less 5-HTP crossed the blood-brain barrier and entered the brain of the depressed subjects than into the brains of the nondepressed controls. This research literally showed evidence that the transport of 5-HTP across the blood-brain barrier may be compromised in people suffering from major depression.

The next question, of course, is whether taking supplemental 5-HTP can help ease depression. Several studies suggest that this is the case. For example, as part of a study done in 1975, Japanese researchers gave 5-HTP to twenty-four patients hospitalized for depression. After two weeks of treatment, they observed a "marked amelioration of depressive symptoms" in seven of the patients. They also found that the use of 5-HTP was associated with a 30 percent increase in the levels of 5-HIAA (the primary metabolite of serotonin) in the participants' cerebrospinal fluid. According to the researchers, these findings suggest that the supplemental 5-HTP was being converted to serotonin in the brain.

Another group of Japanese researchers in 1978 performed a study with fifty-nine patients with depression. They gave the participants between 150 and 300 milligrams of 5-HTP for three weeks. Fully 68 percent improved during the study, and of those 80 percent improved within the first week of treatment.

Studies have also shown that 5-HTP is more effective than tryptophan at improving mood. Double-blind clinical trials have compared the efficacy of tryptophan with that of 5-HTP in the treatment of depression and found the 5-HTP to be clearly superior.

A series of studies dating back to the 1970s have even found 5-HTP to be as effective as tricyclic antidepressants in managing depression. (Tricyclic antidepressants were the class of drugs considered most effective at treating depression until SSRIs like Prozac were introduced.) Researchers found that 5-

HTP was at least as effective as these drugs in treating very severe depression, with fewer side effects.

Other studies have found that 5-HTP can enhance the performance of some traditional antidepressants. For example, a 1976 study found that people treated with the MAO inhibitor antidepressant nialamide along with 5-HTP achieved a fuller recovery than those patients treated with the antidepressant alone. A study done in 1982 found that 5-HTP taken in conjunction with the tricyclic antidepressant clomipramine can give good results in therapy-resistant vital depressions.

COMPARING 5-HTP TO PROZAC

How does 5-HTP measure up against Prozac and the other cutting-edge SSRIs, which are considered the current standard of treatment for depression? The answer came from a ground-breaking double-blind, multicenter study conducted by a team of Swiss and German psychiatric researchers headed by Dr. W. Poeldinger of Switzerland. As part of

the study, sixty-nine participants (all between the ages of eighteen and seventy-five
and all diagnosed with clinical depression)
received either 100 milligrams of 5-HTP three
times a day, or 150 milligrams of fluvoxamine
(the SSRI commonly known as Luvox) three
times a day. The participants were evaluated
before and at two, four, and six weeks into the
study, using standard depression rating
scales (the Hamilton Rating Scale for Depression and a standard psychiatric test). At each
interval, the subjects also evaluated and reported how they felt.

The results offered dramatic evidence of
the effectiveness of 5-HTP. Participants on
both 5-HTP and the SSRI showed a significant
(and nearly equal) reduction in depression
beginning at week two and continuing
through week six. After four weeks, fifteen of
the thirty-six patients taking 5-HTP and eighteen of the thirty-three patients taking the
SSRI had improved by at least 50 percent, using the scores on the depression rating scales
as a relative measure. By week six, both
groups had about equal numbers of people

showing 50 percent improvement. (The participants' self-assessments tracked the scores on the depression rating scales.)

In addition, the 5-HTP tended to produce fewer side effects than the SSRI. Generally speaking, unpleasant side effects were rare and mild for both 5-HTP and the SSRI. In both groups the symptoms tended to appear during the first few days of treatment and then fade away. A review of serious side effects associated with the SSRI from the *Physician's Desk Reference* was extensive, though there are no serious side effects associated with 5-HTP when it is taken at the levels used in the studies conducted by scientists and researchers studying the effects of 5-HTP.

Dr. Poeldinger and his colleagues suggest that 5-HTP may not be treating depression per se, but instead may be treating the much broader problem that underlies the depression. This condition, which they refer to as "serotonin deficiency syndrome," may show up as depression, but it can also take the form of anxiety, insomnia, aggressiveness, migraine headaches, and obsessive-compulsive behaviors, among others. In other words, there is reason to believe that 5-HTP could be successful at treating every medical problem currently being treated using SSRIs.

Why is 5-HTP as effective as SSRIs at treating depression? Poeldinger and colleagues point out that the SSRIs work in a very precise manner by targeting the neurotransmitter serotonin. SSRIs do not affect the other neurotransmitters, specifically noradrenergic (NA) and dopaminergic (DA) pathways.

On the other hand, 5-HTP is somewhat less targeted. It is converted into serotonin not only in serotonergic neurons but also in dopaminergic and noradrenergic neurons. These other neurotransmitters may be involved in the relief of depression, and the 5-HTP ·may act as a false transmitter to stimulate different types of neurotransmission. This may explain why 5-HTP has been found to be as good as or better than both tryptophan and SSRIs as an antidepressant.

ARE YOU DEPRESSED?

At some point in their lives, most people experience depression. In some cases, depression can be relieved through the use of nutritional supplements, such as 5-HTP. Other times, professional assistance may be needed to manage a crisis situation or to prescribe appropriate medication. This section will help you identify the warning signs of depression and to determine if 5-HTP might be helpful in the treatment of the condition.

Everyone feels sadness in response to certain situations—the death of a loved one, the loss of a job, a divorce, or some other disappointment. Depression, on the other hand, is characterized by ongoing feelings of sadness, worthlessness, and lack of interest in life. With clinical depression, these feelings linger for weeks or months and ultimately become incapacitating. Depression can be either a short-term, minor problem or a lifelong, life-threatening illness. In fact, more than four out of five people who commit suicide are depressed.

Some people inherit a tendency to develop depression due to their brain chemistry. Other times the illness is brought on by physical conditions, such as stroke, hepatitis, chronic fatigue syndrome, chronic stress, thyroid disease, menopause, alcoholism, drug abuse, or even the lack of natural light during the darker winter months.

Whatever the cause, most cases of depression involve an imbalance of the neurotransmitters, especially serotonin. Although depression was once considered a shameful psychiatric condition, most experts now recognize that it usually has both physical and psychological triggers. It is an organic illness involving physical, biochemical changes in the body, so without help the person cannot "snap out of it," no matter how hard he or she tries.

It can be difficult to tell the difference between clinical depression and common sadness. But there are certain warning signs, including:

- Changes in sleep, to either insomnia or sleepiness
- Changes in weight and eating habits, either weight gain or weight loss
- Loss of sexual desire or libido
- Chronic fatigue or tiredness
- Low self-esteem or self-worth
- Loss of productivity at work, home, or school
- Inability to concentrate or think clearly
- Withdrawal or isolation
- Loss of interest in activities that were once enjoyable
- Anger or irritability
- Trouble accepting praise or affirmation
- Feeling slow; every activity takes supreme effort
- Apprehension about the future
- Frequent weeping or sobbing
- Thoughts of suicide or death

These are all warning signs and diagnostic criteria for depression. If you or a loved one experiences three or more of these symptoms for two weeks or longer, contact a doctor or mental health professional for help. Don't try to treat serious depression by yourself. If you or someone you're concerned about feels suicidal, immediately seek help from a specialist or a twenty-four-hour hot line; look in the Yellow Pages under "Suicide Prevention."

On the other hand, 5-HTP can be helpful in improving mild depression or prolonged sadness. In addition, you may be able to prevent some episodes of depression—as well as generally elevate your mood—by getting regular exercise and rest and by sharing your feelings with someone you trust. Be aware that depression and sadness can also be side effects of many medications, including over-the-counter antihistamines. If you suspect that your mood changes are drug induced, talk to your doctor about the medications you are taking.

ARE YOU DEPRESSED OR JUST FEELING BLUE?

If you want an accurate assessment of your state of mind, you can take this test known as the CES-D (Center for Epidemiological Studies—Depression). It was developed by Lenore Radloff at the National Institute of Mental Health. For each item, mark the choice that best describes how you have felt over the past week.

1. *I was bothered by things that usually don't bother me.*

   0 Rarely or none of the time (less than one day)
   1 Some or a little of the time (one to two days)
   2 Occasionally or a moderate amount of the time (three or four days)
   3 Most or all of the time (five to seven days)

2. *I did not feel like eating; my appetite was poor.*

   0 Rarely or none of the time (less than one day)
   1 Some or a little of the time (one to two days)
   2 Occasionally or a moderate amount of the time (three or four days)
   3 Most or all of the time (five to seven days)

3. *I felt that I could not shake off the blues even with help from my family and friends.*

   0 Rarely or none of the time (less than one day)
   1 Some or a little of the time (one to two days)
   2 Occasionally or a moderate amount of the time (three or four days)
   3 Most or all of the time (five to seven days)

4. *I felt that I was not as good as other people.*

   0 Rarely or none of the time (less than one day)

   1 Some or a little of the time (one to two days)

   2 Occasionally or a moderate amount of the time (three or four days)

   3 Most or all of the time (five to seven days)

5. *I had trouble keeping my mind on what I was doing.*

   0 Rarely or none of the time (less than one day)

   1 Some or a little of the time (one to two days)

   2 Occasionally or a moderate amount of the time (three or four days)

   3 Most or all of the time (five to seven days)

6. *I felt depressed.*

   0 Rarely or none of the time (less than one day)

   1 Some or a little of the time (one to two days)

   2 Occasionally or a moderate amount of the time (three or four days)

   3 Most or all of the time (five to seven days)

7. *I felt that everything I did was an effort.*

   0 Rarely or none of the time (less than one day)
   1 Some or a little of the time (one to two days)
   2 Occasionally or a moderate amount of the time (three or four days)
   3 Most or all of the time (five to seven days)

8. *I felt hopeless about the future.*

   0 Rarely or none of the time (less than one day)
   1 Some or a little of the time (one to two days)
   2 Occasionally or a moderate amount of the time (three or four days)
   3 Most or all of the time (five to seven days)

9. *I thought my life had been a failure.*

   0 Rarely or none of the time (less than one day)
   1 Some or a little of the time (one to two days)
   2 Occasionally or a moderate amount of the time (three or four days)
   3 Most or all of the time (five to seven days)

10. *I felt fearful.*

   0 Rarely or none of the time (less than one day)
   1 Some or a little of the time (one to two days)

2 Occasionally or a moderate amount of the time (three or four days)

3 Most or all of the time (five to seven days)

11. *My sleep was restless.*

0 Rarely or none of the time (less than one day)
1 Some or a little of the time (one to two days)
2 Occasionally or a moderate amount of the time (three or four days)
3 Most or all of the time (five to seven days)

12. *I was unhappy.*

0 Rarely or none of the time (less than one day)
1 Some or a little of the time (one to two days)
2 Occasionally or a moderate amount of the time (three or four days)
3 Most or all of the time (five to seven days)

13. *I talked less than usual.*

0 Rarely or none of the time (less than one day)
1 Some or a little of the time (one to two days)
2 Occasionally or a moderate amount of the time (three or four days)
3 Most or all of the time (five to seven days)

14. *I felt lonely.*

   0 Rarely or none of the time (less than one day)
   1 Some or a little of the time (one to two days)
   2 Occasionally or a moderate amount of the
      time (three or four days)
   3 Most or all of the time (five to seven days)

15. *People were unfriendly.*

   0 Rarely or none of the time (less than one day)
   1 Some or a little of the time (one to two days)
   2 Occasionally or a moderate amount of the
      time (three or four days)
   3 Most or all of the time (five to seven days)

16. *I did not enjoy life.*

   0 Rarely or none of the time (less than one day)
   1 Some or a little of the time (one to two days)
   2 Occasionally or a moderate amount of the
      time (three or four days)
   3 Most or all of the time (five to seven days)

17. *I had crying spells.*

   0 Rarely or none of the time (less than one day)
   1 Some or a little of the time (one to two days)

2 Occasionally or a moderate amount of the
time (three or four days)

3 Most or all of the time (five to seven days)

18. *I felt sad.*

0 Rarely or none of the time (less than one day)

1 Some or a little of the time (one to two days)

2 Occasionally or a moderate amount of the
time (three or four days)

3 Most or all of the time (five to seven days)

19. *I felt that people dislike me.*

0 Rarely or none of the time (less than one day)

1 Some or a little of the time (one to two days)

2 Occasionally or a moderate amount of the
time (three or four days)

3 Most or all of the time (five to seven days)

20. *I could not get "going."*

0 Rarely or none of the time (less than one day)

1 Some or a little of the time (one to two days)

2 Occasionally or a moderate amount of the
time (three or four days)

3 Most or all of the time (five to seven days)

Tally your score by adding up the numbers
you circled. If your score was 22 or higher,
you may be suffering from major depression
and should seek professional care. If your
score was 15 to 21, you may be experiencing
mild depression and may find 5-HTP helpful
in easing your symptoms.

ARE YOU A CANDIDATE FOR 5-HTP?

After reading the information in this chapter,
do you suspect that you are suffering from
mild depression? If so, you may want to try
using 5-HTP to improve your mood. While 5-
HTP can be effective at easing major depression, you should be under professional care
if you have reason to believe your depression
is more severe. (For more information on using the supplement, see Chapter 6, "The Safe
and Effective Use of 5-HTP.")

While you may find a boost in mood immediately after taking 5-HTP, it may take several weeks for your body to adjust and for the depression to lift. If the symptoms of depression do not respond to 5-HTP within two to three weeks, please consult your doctor or another medical professional for assistance. The resources listed at the end of this chapter may also prove useful.

WARNING: Do not take 5-HTP if you are already taking prescription drugs to treat your depression. The combination of 5-HTP and antidepressants can be dangerous. If you are interested in taking 5-HTP and are currently taking any form of antidepressants, discuss the matter with your doctor.

CALL FOR HELP

American Psychiatric Association
Division of Public Affairs
(202) 682-6220
This group can provide referrals to psychiatrists in your area who specialize in treating depression.

TYPES OF DEPRESSION

There are two main types of depression: unipolar and bipolar depression. Unipolar depression involves depression alone, or the feelings of exhaustion and withdrawal from activities and involvement. Bipolar depression involves mood swings between depression and manic behavior. Manic behavior involves violent, aggressive physical activity, restlessness, and the feeling of being mentally supercharged. Together, these conditions are known as affective disorders.

Depression Awareness, Recognition, and Treatment (D/ART)
(800) 421-4211

Depression and Related Affective Disorders Association
Johns Hopkins Hospital
600 North Wolfe Street
Baltimore, MD 21287
(410) 955-4647

Depressives Anonymous: Recovering from Depression
329 East 62 Street
New York, NY 10021
(212) 689-2600

Foundation for Depression and Manic Depression
24 East 81 Street, Suite 2B
New York, NY 10028
(212) 772-3400

National Alliance for the Mentally Ill
200 North Glebe Road, Suite 1015
Arlington, VA 22203-3754
(800) 950-6264

National Depressive and Manic Depressive Association
730 North Franklin Street, Suite 501
Chicago, IL 60610
(312) 642-0049
(800) 826-3632

National Foundation for Depressive Illness
P.O. Box 2257
New York, NY 10116
(212) 268-4260

National Mental Health Association
1021 Prince Street
Alexandria, VA 22314
(703) 684-7722
(800) 243-2525

4. SATISFY YOUR *REAL* CRAVINGS: 5-HTP AND EATING DISORDERS

WHEN A CRAVING STRIKES, IT CAN BE ALL-consuming. No matter what you do or where you go to escape the urge, you just can't shake your obsession for that slice of Black Forest layer cake or that bag of nacho-flavored chips. Resisting the desire takes enormous amounts of energy; giving in to the desire offers a moment of ecstasy, followed by guilt, anger, and self-loathing. You may be left wondering, Why can't I control my eating?

While our eating patterns involve a complex range of physical, social, and emotional factors, our cravings and culinary desires also reflect our brain chemistry. Once again, the neurotransmitter serotonin appears to be one of the most critical factors controlling appetite.

Our biochemical response to food is triggered before we lift a fork. In fact, the sight, the smell, or even the anticipation of food stimulates the release of serotonin in the hypothalamus, a tiny part of the brain that oversees our eating and sleeping habits. Once we begin to eat, the serotonin levels continue to rise; when serotonin levels reach a critical level, the hypothalamus sends out messages that your stomach is full and your craving has been satisfied. In other words, you stop eating when your brain says you're full, not when your stomach says you're full.

As you might imagine, problems can arise when serotonin levels are insufficient, leaving the body with a diminished capacity to experience satiety or satisfaction after a meal. Of course, a number of other neurotransmitters play a role in orchestrating appetite and food intake, but serotonin appears to oversee the process. In fact, researchers have shown that you can decrease food consumption by increasing serotonin activity in the brain; conversely, you can increase food consumption by decreasing serotonin activity in the brain.

Research done on animals dramatically demonstrates the importance of the hypothalamus in controlling eating behavior. When researchers destroyed one area of the hypothalamus, the animals refused to consume any food and water; when they damaged another portion, the animals ate without stopping, as though they were unable to turn off the signal for hunger. Of course, research done on animals in a laboratory does not directly reflect human behavior in the real world, but it does suggest that eating disorders—including both the extremes of overeating and self-starvation—may be influenced by problems with the hypothalamus.

A review of ten years of research on serotonin and appetite concludes that serotonin may be responsible for controlling appetite and eating habits. University of Leeds researcher John Blundell notes that the human digestive tract is replete with serotonin receptors, which may be designed to gauge the body's nutritional requirements and provide constant feedback to trigger feelings of hunger and satiety.

SEROTONIN AND EATING DISORDERS

Most people crave carbohydrates and other foods from time to time, but cravings sometimes get out of control, resulting in an eating disorder such as bulimia nervosa (bingeing and purging) or compulsive overeating (bingeing without purging) or even anorexia nervosa (self-starvation).

A study published in the *American Journal of Psychiatry* in 1995 found that women with bulimia nervosa have an exaggerated or pathological response to changes in serotonin activity. In one experiment, researchers tested this hypothesis by feeding women a diet free of tryptophan to see how they would respond. The bulimic women in the study consumed

ARE CARBOHYDRATES WHAT YOU CRAVE?

Ice cream, milk, cookies, candy, chocolate, peanut butter, bread, cereal, muffins, macaroni and cheese, pretzels, chips, and popcorn. You choose your favorites, but chances are good that your shopping list includes these and other favorite high-carbohydrate foods when you're lost in a food binge.

You may be using food to improve your mood. That binge may be triggered by low levels of serotonin in your brain, and you may be self-medicating with food to soothe your mood by raising your serotonin levels. In the body, carbohydrates temporarily raise serotonin activity, providing a brief—but real—boost in mood and feeling of calm during and after a binge. This is one reason people tend to crave carbohydrates (especially sugar and starch) when they're under stress.

Unfortunately, binge eating can result in weight problems, nutritional imbalances, and psychological stress associated with a behavior perceived as shameful. You can, however, minimize binge eating and maintain a more balanced approach to eating by sustaining healthy levels of serotonin in the brain. The nutritional supplement 5-HTP can be helpful in curbing cravings and overcoming eating disorders. (For more information on using 5-HTP, see Chapter 6, ''The Safe and Effective Use of 5-HTP.'')

more calories and experienced more irritability and mood disturbance when denied tryptophan than did women who did not suffer from an eating disorder. The researchers concluded that bulimics may be more vulnerable to shifts of tryptophan availability and serotonin levels, which may trigger episodes of binge eating.

Ironically, the same brain chemical that can cause binge eating can also cause anorexia nervosa, or self-starvation. However, studies show that anorexia may be the manifestation of an overactive rather than an underactive serotonin system.

Dr. Walter Kaye and his colleagues at the University of Pittsburgh believe that people suffering from anorexia may have a hyperactive serotonin system that forces them to be self-controlled to the point of dysfunction. (In addition to starving themselves, anorexics tend to be perfectionistic, rigid, and inhibited.)

Since serotonin triggers a feeling of fullness and diminishes the desire for eating, people with high serotonin activity might not feel hungry as often as people with normal serotonin activity, and they may feel satisfied after eating just a few bites of food. In essence, people with anorexia may be self-medicating by denying themselves food to lower their serotonin levels, just as people with bulimia consume large quantities of food to raise their serotonin levels. Anorexics report that they feel better when they refuse to eat, just as bulimics report that they feel better when they binge. In other words, bulimia and anorexia appear to be opposite expressions of the same problem—an imbalance of serotonin in the brain.

Several studies have determined that anorexics have higher levels of serotonin metabolite in their spinal fluid, indicating that they may be experiencing a higher than normal level of serotonin activity. This holds true both during their periods of fasting and purging and after they have reached a healthy goal weight after treatment, which may explain why anorexia is often a lifetime struggle.

WHAT ABOUT REDUX?

Because of the apparent link between serotonin and eating disorders, many doctors and nutrition experts have looked to prescription drugs designed to alter serotonin levels to help control binge eating and other eating disorders. None of the SSRIs has proven consistently reliable at treating eating disorders, though Prozac often (but not always) helps compulsive overeaters reduce their number of binge eating sessions, and it can suppress the appetite in some people.

One exception was the antiobesity drug Redux (dexfenfluramine), which was approved by the FDA, then withdrawn from the market in 1997 when it was found to cause heart valve problems in some patients. Redux alters serotonin activity in the brain, but there is a critical difference between Redux and Prozac and the other SSRIs. The SSRIs allow serotonin to circulate in the brain for a longer period of time so that the brain can maximize the benefits associated with the serotonin produced by the body. Redux, on the other hand, forces the nerve cells to produce higher levels of serotonin and then allows that superdose of serotonin to circulate longer. The serious complications associated with Redux may have been caused by overdosing the neurons with serotonin and essentially burning them out. New evidence suggests that as many as 30 percent of Redux users could develop abnormalities in the shape of their heart valves, which could lead to serious cardiac complications.

Millions of Americans used Redux to help them lose weight. While Redux is no longer available, there is an effective and safe alternative. The nutrition supplement 5-HTP offers the same serotonin-raising benefits as Redux, without the side effects.

USING 5-HTP TO CONTROL YOUR CRAVINGS

Research shows that 5-HTP can help control food cravings and overeating. Obesity and compulsive overeating have been linked to serotonin deficiency, so it follows that balancing serotonin levels should help control feelings of hunger and craving. Taking the nutritional supplement 5-HTP can short-circuit this overpowering desire to eat, allowing you to control your appetite and limit your eating.

Research indicates that 5-HTP may provide many of the same appetite control benefits as SSRIs. According to a 1992 article in the *American Journal of Clinical Nutrition*, 5-HTP can be used safely to treat obesity, with few (if any) side effects. A group of Italian researchers gave twenty obese patients 900 milligrams of 5-HTP a day; the study participants lost a significant amount of weight, craved fewer carbohydrates, and consistently became satisfied with less food than a similar group taking a placebo.

Other studies show that 5-HTP helps with cravings and eating disorders at much lower doses. According to a study reported in the *American Journal of Clinical Nutrition*, 5-HTP is an effective appetite suppressant at low doses (50 to 100 milligrams) if taken a half hour before meals. During a six-week clinical trial using obese subjects, participants who took 5-HTP at these levels voluntarily decreased their caloric intake of both carbohydrates and fats, but not protein. The people in the study lost a significant amount of weight because they cut calories on their own, not because they were on any kind of a restricted diet.

A PRIMER ON EATING DISORDERS

If you suspect that you or someone you know has an eating disorder, you may want to discuss using 5-HTP with your physician. While eating habits can be a very personal matter, it is important to recognize the symptoms of eating disorders so that you can seek treatment, if needed. This section identifies the symptoms of the most common types of eating disorders.

Anorexia Nervosa

Anorexia nervosa is identified by the following criteria:

- The person is not satisfied with a body weight that is at least 15 percent below the minimal normal weight for his or her age and height.

- The person experiences intense fear of gaining weight or becoming fat, even though he or she is grossly underweight.

- The person has a distorted body image or perception of body weight, size, or shape. He or she may claim to feel fat even when emaciated, or argue that one area of the body is too fat even when it is obviously underweight.

- In females, a woman misses at least three consecutive menstrual cycles that were expected to occur (this condition is known as amenorrhea).

As a result of the illness, people suffering from anorexia starve themselves to the point of emaciation—or death. In fact, 10 to 15 percent of people with anorexia nervosa die as a result of their illness.

Anorexia nervosa afflicts females most of the time, usually starting during adolescence or early adulthood. It appears to be a growing problem; in some studies the prevalence of anorexia nervosa has been reported to be as high as one in ninety adolescent girls. The severity and duration of the condition can vary widely. For some anorexics, the condition disappears spontaneously after a few weeks or months. For most anorexics, however, the condition is a chronic, lifelong struggle that can be life-threatening without treatment.

Bulimia Nervosa

Bulimia nervosa is identified by the following criteria:

- The person experiences repeated episodes of binge eating, rapid consumption of a large amount of food in a short period of time.

- The person feels a complete lack of control over his or her eating behavior during the binges.

- The person regularly purges to rid the body of the excess food. The person may rely on self-induced vomiting, laxatives or diuretics, strict dieting or fasting, or vigorous exercise in order to prevent weight gain.

- The person experiences a minimum average of two binge-eating episodes a week for at least three months.

- The person is chronically obsessed with body shape and weight.

During an episode of bingeing, the bulimic gorges on an extraordinary amount of food, often junk food. After gobbling down the food, the bulimic purges to get rid of the food and to avoid gaining weight. Although the numbers vary widely, bulimics usually binge and purge at least once a day, with the average being twelve times a week.

Bulimia is much more common in females, although a growing number of male bulimics are being identified. In various population studies of high school and college students, the prevalence of bulimia nervosa has ranged from 8 percent to 20 percent of the female population and as high as 1.4 percent of the male population.

While some bulimics can hide their symptoms and carry on relatively normal lives, many become incapacitated by their eating disorder. In severe cases, people with bulimia experience an electrolyte imbalance (brought on by the vomiting and use of laxatives), which can result in death due to cardiac arrhythmia. In addition, repeated vomiting sometimes results in rupture of the esophagus, and excessive bingeing has even been known to rupture the stomach.

Others

There are other eating disorders that do not meet the full criteria for anorexia nervosa or bulimia, including

- A person of average weight who does not binge but often self-induces vomiting for fear of gaining weight.
- A female who exhibits all of the features of anorexia nervosa except the absence of menstruation.
- A person who exhibits all of the features of bulimia nervosa except for the frequency of binge-eating episodes.

Compulsive Overeating

For people who suffer from compulsive over-eating, eating becomes an overpowering and inescapable obsession. These people can consume thousands of calories at a sitting, as they devour huge quantities of food. They cannot control their eating, and an episode of bingeing is often followed by excruciating self-loathing and feelings of disgust.

Compulsive overeating is not considered a clinical condition by all members of the medical establishment. Yet millions of Americans recognize their dysfunctional eating behavior as compulsive overeating.

Compulsive overeating is a disease that involves frequent bingeing on enormous amounts of food, often to combat stress. Many compulsive overeaters are overweight, frequently to the point of obesity (20 to 30 percent over their appropriate weight). The obesity can lead to heart disease, high blood pressure, diabetes, bone and joint disease, and other conditions associated with being overweight.

Compulsive overeating occurs in both men and women. It often begins during childhood or adolescence, although it also can develop later in life. Accurate statistics regarding the prevalence of compulsive overeating are not available, but it is obviously a serious problem among Americans.

Many compulsive overeaters—and many people with other eating disorders—tend to experience depression. They may feel hopelessness or worthlessness, and as they fail in their efforts to control their eating disorder, they may be increasingly self-critical. Thoughts and feelings of suicide (as well as suicide attempts) are relatively common among people with eating disorders.

FOOD ADDICTION

Many people who struggle with eating disorders know from firsthand experience that food can be addictive. In many cases, people use food to alter their brain chemistry to produce a high.

In much the same way that we eat to alter our serotonin levels, some people increase their serotonin levels by using addictive substances such as alcohol, caffeine, tobacco, and certain narcotics. If a person tries to stop using any of these addictive substances, a chemical withdrawal syndrome occurs when serotonin levels plummet. This supports the notion that overeating is, in part, a chemical dependency caused by low serotonin levels, and that a person can be addicted to Twinkies in much the same way he or she can be addicted to cigarettes or heroin.

This concept of food addiction is the basis of the Overeaters Anonymous approach to overcoming eating disorders. Overeaters Anonymous and other support groups can provide a network of support during the process of overcoming an eating disorder. In many cases, people become psychologically addicted to food, even though the problem may have had biological roots. Following are the twelve steps of the Overeaters Anonymous program; for information on contacting the organization, see page 88.

1. We admitted we were powerless over food—that our lives had become unmanageable.

2. Came to believe that a power greater than ourselves could restore us to sanity.

3. Made a decision to turn our will and our lives over to the care of God *as we understood Him.*

4. Made a searching and fearless moral inventory of ourselves.

5. Admitted to God, to ourselves, and to another human being the exact nature of our wrongs.

6. Were entirely ready to have God remove all these defects of character.

7. Humbly asked Him to remove our shortcomings.

8. Made a list of all persons we had harmed, and became willing to make amends to them all.

9. Made direct amends to such people wherever possible, except when to do so would injure them or others,

10. Continued to take personal inventory and when we were wrong, promptly admitted it.

11. Sought through prayer and meditation to improve our conscious contact with God

as we understood Him, praying only for
knowledge of His will for us and the
power to carry that out.

12. Having had a spiritual awakening as the
result of these steps, we tried to carry this
message to compulsive overeaters and to
practice these principles in all our affairs.

ARE YOU A CANDIDATE FOR 5-HTP?

If you believe that you may be suffering from
an eating disorder, you may want to ask your
physician about using 5-HTP to regain control over your eating and to establish more
healthful eating patterns. (For more information on using the nutritional supplement, see
Chapter 6, "The Safe and Effective Use of 5-
HTP.")

As the research presented in this chapter
shows, 5-HTP can be effective at treating even
severe eating problems. However, if you are
suffering from clinical anorexia nervosa or
bulimia nervosa (as defined in this chapter),
please seek professional medical care. Eating
disorders that have progressed to an advanced stage can be difficult to treat and re-

quire expert assistance. In addition, you may want to contact some of the organizations listed below for more information on eating disorders in general.

CALL FOR HELP

The following organizations and associations can provide further information on eating disorders.

American Anorexia/Bulimia Association (AABA)
133 Cedar Lane
Teaneck, NJ 07666
(201) 863-1800

American Dietetic Association
216 W. Jackson Blvd.
Suite 800
Chicago, IL 60606
(312) 899-0040

Anorexia and Bulimia Resource Center
2699 South Bayshore, Suite 800-E
Coconut Grove, FL 33133
(305) 854-0652

Anorexia and Bulimia Treatment and Education Center
(800) 33-ABTEC
(301) 332-9800 in Maryland

Anorexia Nervosa and Related Eating Disorders, Inc.
P.O. Box 5102
Eugene, OR 97405
(503) 344-1144

Breaking Free Seminars (Compulsive Overeating)
Expo Associates
452 Eston Road
Wellesley, MA 02181
(617) 431-7807

Center for the Study of Anorexia and Bulimia
1 West 91 Street
New York, NY 10024
(212) 595-3449

Eating Disorders Center
330 West 58 Street, Suite 200
New York, NY 10019
(212) 582-1345

Food and Drug Administration
Office of Consumer Affairs
5600 Fishers Lane
HFE-88
Rockville, MD 20857
(301) 443-3170

Food and Nutrition Information Center
National Agricultural Library
Room 304
Beltsville, MD 20705
(301) 344-3719

National Anorexia Aid Society
The Bridge Foundation
5796 Karl Road
Columbus, OH 43229
(614) 436-1112
(614) 846-2833

**National Association of Anorexia Nervosa
and Associated Disorders**
Box 7
Highland Park, IL 60035
(312) 831-3438

**National Cholesterol Education Program
Information Center**
4733 Bethesda Avenue, Room 530
Bethesda, MD 20814
(301) 951-3260

**National Eating Disorder Information
Center**
1560 Bayview Avenue, Suite 203
Toronto, Ontario
Canada M4G 388
(416) 483-5219

Overeaters Anonymous
World Service Office
4025 Spencer Street, #203
Torrance, CA 90503
(310) 542-8363

Weight Loss/Behavior Modification Program for Teens
Shapedown
Balboa Publishing
101 Larkspur Landing
Larkspur, CA 94939
(415) 453-8886

Some Leading Eating Disorders Clinics

Alabama
University of Alabama
Weight Reduction and Eating Disorders Center
Department of Nutrition Sciences
WEBB 212
Birmingham, AL 35294
(205) 934-5112

Arizona
University of Arizona Health Sciences Center
Eating Disorders Program
Tucson, AZ 85724
(602) 626-6509

California
University of California
Eating Disorders Clinic
Neuropsychiatric Institute
Los Angeles, CA 90024
(213) 825-0173

District of Columbia
George Washington University Medical
Center
Eating Disorders Clinic
2150 Pennsylvania Avenue, NW
Washington, DC 20037
(202) 994-1000
(202) 676-8298

Florida
University of South Florida
College of Medicine
Eating Disorders Clinic
12901 North 30 Street
Box 14
Tampa, FL 33612
(813) 974-4242

Georgia
Emory University Woodruff Health Sciences
Center
Parkwood Hospital
Eating Disorders Clinic
Atlanta, GA 30322
(404) 321-0111

Illinois
Northwestern University
Northwestern Memorial Hospital
Eating Disorders Clinic
Chicago, IL 60611
(312) 908-8100

Iowa
University of Iowa Psychiatric Hospital
Eating Disorders Clinic
Iowa City, IA 52242
(319) 353-3719

Kentucky
Eating Disorders Recognition and
Intervention Program
Norton Psychiatric Clinic

P.O. Box 35070
Louisville, KY 40232
(502) 562-8853

Louisiana
Tulane University Hospital
Eating Disorders Program
New Orleans, LA 70112
(504) 588-5405

Maryland
The Johns Hopkins University
Eating and Weight Disorder Clinic
Baltimore, MD 21205
(301) 955-5514

Massachusetts
Frances Stern Nutrition Center
Tufts University School of Medicine
New England Medical Center
171 Harrison Avenue
Boston, MA 02111
(617) 726-3588

Michigan
University of Michigan Medical Center
Eating Disorders Clinic
Ann Arbor, MI 48109
(313) 764-0210

Minnesota
University of Minnesota Hospital and Clinic
Anorexia Nervosa and Bulimia Treatment
Program
Box 393 UMHC
Minneapolis, MN 55455
(612) 626-6188

Mississippi
University of Mississippi Medical Center
Eating Disorders Program
Jackson, MS 39216
(601) 984-5805

Nebraska
University of Nebraska Hospital and Clinic
Eating Disorders Program
Omaha, NE 68105
(402) 559-5524

New York
Eating Disorders Clinic
Albert Einstein College of Medicine/
Montefiore Medical Center
Bronx, NY 10467
(212) 920-6613

North Carolina
East Carolina University School of Medicine
Eating Disorders
Psychiatric Medicine
Greenville, NC 27834
(919) 757-2666

Ohio
University of Cincinnati Medical Center
Eating Disorders Center
231 Bethesda Avenue
Cincinnati, OH 45267-0559
(513) 872-5118

Pennsylvania
Eating Disorder Service
Center for Behavioral Medicine
Hospital of the University of Pennsylvania

36 and Spruce Streets
Philadelphia, PA 19104
(215) 662-3503

Texas
University of Texas Health Science Center
Eating Disorders Clinic
5323 Harry Hines Boulevard
Dallas, TX 75235
(214) 688-2218

Utah
University of Utah School of Medicine
Eating Disorders Clinic
50 North Medical Drive
Salt Lake City, UT 84132
(801) 581-8989

Virginia
Medical College of Virginia
Eating Disorders Program
MCV Station
Box 710
Richmond, VA 23298
(804) 786-9157
(804) 786-0762

Wisconsin
University of Wisconsin Hospital and
Clinics
Eating Disorders Program
Madison, WI 53706
(608) 263-6406

5. ALMOST A MIRACLE: 5-HTP AND OTHER HEALTH PROBLEMS

IN ADDITION TO DEPRESSION AND EATING DISorders, a number of emotional and physical problems have been linked to serotonin deficiency syndrome. Because the nutritional supplement 5-HTP can boost serotonin levels naturally, it should come as no surprise to learn that 5-HTP is often quite effective at treating these problems. In fact, 5-HTP can be helpful in the treatment of many of the same problems that SSRIs and other serotonin-active drugs are used to treat.

A survey of the medical literature shows

that 5-HTP has been proved effective in the treatment of a range of medical and mental problems. This chapter provides a summary of a number of conditions that respond well to 5-HTP. Keep in mind, however, that 5-HTP may be used to treat conditions not mentioned here, such as premenstrual syndrome, obsessive-compulsive disorder, and compulsive gambling, among others. The sections included here cover only topics for which there were several articles published in peer-reviewed medical journals providing evidence of the effectiveness of 5-HTP.

If you suffer from a medical condition or syndrome that is linked to serotonin activity (or that involves problems with impulse control), you might want to discuss taking 5-HTP with your physician and see if your symptoms ease, provided you do not fall into one of the categories of people who should not take 5-HTP. (For more information on who should and shouldn't take 5-HTP, see Chapter 6, "The Safe and Effective Use of 5-HTP.")

Many of the conditions discussed in the

chapter are serious health problems that require the attention of a medical professional. *The use of 5-HTP is not intended to replace or substitute for professional care.* Discuss your overall treatment plan with your doctor and ask whether 5-HTP can be used as part of your strategy for health. If you want more information about a specific medical condition discussed in this chapter, please refer to the resources listed in the "Call for Help" section at the end of each entry.

ADDICTION/SUBSTANCE ABUSE

A person suffering from addiction is completely myopic: The world shrinks to a single vision, a single obsession, a single physical yearning. In such cases, the addict longs for— and would do almost anything to receive— the substance he or she is craving. Over time, the cravings may become all-consuming; the perceived need for the drug may surpass the need for food, shelter, relationships, even personal safety.

The real object of desire in many cases of

addiction is not the drug itself but the serotonin rush that follows taking the drug. Some illegal drugs—including Ecstasy (MMDA), cocaine, and some hallucinogens—produce their high by stimulating serotonin activity in the brain. For example, researchers believe that cocaine acts as a serotonin reuptake blocker (using the same mechanism as the prescription drugs known as SSRIs), and that hallucinogenic LSD and "magic mushrooms" (psilocybin) contain compounds that so closely resemble serotonin that they can fit into the serotonin receptors in the neurons. Of course, the biochemical drug reactions are more complex than this, but the point remains that these drugs have a profound influence on serotonin levels and activity.

People with a substance abuse problem often have low levels of serotonin activity, which may explain why they are attracted to and easily become addicted to drugs. One theory is that the low serotonin levels make it more difficult for the individual to exercise impulse control. Another theory is that the depression, anxiety, and other mood disorders associated with low serotonin levels may be an underlying cause of the drug use.

A study published in the *American Journal of Psychiatry* in 1983 found that the nutritional supplement 5-HTP helped to reverse the symptoms of a twenty-three-year-old man suffering from LSD-induced psychosis. This research supports the idea that some LSD-induced psychotic disorders may be caused by a deficiency of serotonin.

Other studies in both animals and humans have shown than 5-HTP and some serotonin-active drugs can reduce cravings for drugs. However, the amount of improvement varies dramatically from individual to individual.

Still, the research is promising enough that if you or someone you know uses drugs and wants to stop, the nutritional supplement 5-HTP may be able to help take an edge off of the cravings and impulsive behavior. (For information on using 5-HTP, see Chapter 6, "The Safe and Effective Use of 5-HTP.")

CALL FOR HELP

Center for Substance Abuse Prevention
(800) 843-4971

Cocaine Anonymous
(800) COCAINE
(213) 559-5833

The Hazelden Foundation
(800) I-DO-CARE

Johnson Institute
(800) 247-0484
(800) 231-5165 in Minnesota

Narcotics Anonymous
(800) 662-4357
(818) 780-3951

National Institute on Alcoholism and Drug Dependence
(212) 206-6770

Rational Recovery
(916) 621-4374

Secular Organizations for Sobriety (SOS)
(716) 834-2922

ALCOHOLISM

Alcoholism does not discriminate: It destroys individuals and families of every age, race, and socioeconomic class. Its devastating effects can be seen in inner-city slums and in pricey penthouse apartments, in the faces of the dispossessed and unemployed and the faces of powerful and privileged executives. In fact, twenty million Americans are alcohol dependent or drink enough to be at risk of impaired health.

Although the cause and the physiology of alcoholism have been debated over the years, research suggests that alcoholism may be triggered by low levels of serotonin in the brain. In fact, many people use alcohol to self-medicate during times they feel stressed or anxious. This behavior makes sense because drinking temporarily raises serotonin levels, but it then causes serotonin levels to crash, reinforcing the desire to drink again.

The depression and mood disorders associated with low serotonin levels can also trigger the desire for alcohol. In addition, the low serotonin levels can make it more difficult for a person to resist the impulse to drink alcohol. In other words, the craving is strong, the impulse control is weak, and the person may have little ability to resist drinking.

While alcohol acts on the central nervous system in a number of ways, it tends to affect behaviors regulated by the serotonin system. For example, alcohol relaxes mood or sedates, loosen inhibitions, suppresses pain, and depresses motor control.

Alcoholism is a difficult problem to overcome in part because drinking alcohol does provide the serotonin rush that is so rewarding to the drinker. By measuring the levels of serotonin metabolites in the urine and blood after a single drinking session, researchers have learned that alcohol triggers an increase in serotonin release in the nervous system. However, a number of animal studies indicate that long-term, chronic drinking actually impairs serotonin activity, rather than stimulating it, which may promote additional drinking.

Some fascinating research has been done on serotonin and alcoholism using rats. The animals were bred for alcohol preference or nonpreference. When the researchers looked at the concentrations of neurotransmitters in different parts of the rat brains, they found that the levels of serotonin and its metabolites were lower in those rats that preferred alcohol, as compared to the "normal" rats that did not prefer alcohol. Some researchers have gone on to hypothesize that alcoholism and heavy drinking may be attempts to raise serotonin levels in the brain.

Studies have shown that 5-HTP can be helpful in reinforcing resistance to drinking alcohol. A study done in 1978 allowed rats to have access to either distilled water or a 2 percent solution of ethanol as their only fluid during a one-hour period daily. When 5-HTP was given one hour before the drinking sessions, those rats that took the 5-HTP drank significantly less alcohol than the rats that didn't receive 5-HTP. However, the protective effect and the improved willpower last only a half hour to an hour after taking the 5-HTP.

5-HTP also appears helpful during withdrawal from alcohol. An article published in 1975 in the *American Journal of Psychiatry* suggests that an alcoholic experiences an even greater decrease in serotonin levels during withdrawal, but that 5-HTP partially offsets this problem by raising serotonin levels. Animal studies have found that serotonin activity drops when chronic drinking stops, which may be another reason why quitting can be so difficult and stressful.

5-HTP and other treatments to enhance serotonin activity have been shown to decrease alcohol consumption in laboratory rats by as much as 50 percent. The results on humans are not as clear-cut, but evidence certainly indicates that 5-HTP should help people reduce their cravings for alcohol.

Since alcoholism is a multifaceted addiction that involves emotional and psychological factors as well as physical cravings, merely correcting the serotonin imbalance does not overcome the addiction. However, balancing serotonin levels may help the individual resist the craving for alcohol. If you drink more than you think you should, ask your physician about the possible use of 5-HTP since research shows that it may cut your craving for alcohol. (For more information on using 5-HTP, see Chapter 6, "The Safe and Effective Use of 5-HTP.") In addition, your chances of success improve if you seek professional help from one of the groups listed below.

CALL FOR HELP

Alcoholics Anonymous
(212) 870-3400
Or check Yellow Pages for local listing

The Hazelden Foundation
(800) I-DO-CARE

Johnson Institute
(800) 247-0484
(800) 231-5165 in Minnesota

WHAT IS AN ALCOHOLIC?

An alcoholic is someone who cannot consume alcohol in moderation. Alcoholism may be triggered by a genetic predisposition, a metabolic problem, an allergy, or an imbalance of serotonin in the brain.

Alcohol is a toxin that systematically destroys the body. Alcohol inhibits the liver's production of digestive enzymes and interferes with the body's ability to absorb vitamins A, B, D, E, and K. Alcohol irritates the lining of the gastrointestinal tract, including the esophagus, stomach, and upper small intestine. It increases the production of hydrochloric acid in the stomach, causing inflammation and abdominal pain. It also crosses the blood-brain barrier and damages brain tissues, sometimes resulting in psychological or behavioral problems.

Alcoholism can cause painful nerve inflammation or a condition known as polyneuritis. (This is especially common when there is a deficiency in B vitamins.) Alcohol contributes to diabetes and hypoglycemia because the chronic use can weaken glucose tolerance.

National Clearinghouse for Alcohol and Drug Information
(301) 468-2600

HOW MUCH IS TOO MUCH?

If you consume enough alcohol on a regular basis, it will damage your body—period. Drinking 80 grams of alcohol—a 6-pack of beer, five 6-ounce glasses of wine, or five martinis—is enough to damage the liver and pancreas. The liver is affected because it is the only organ that metabolizes alcohol. (Fully 95 percent of alcohol is metabolized by the liver; the remaining 5 percent is excreted through sweat, urine, and breathing.) In the body, alcohol is converted into fat rather than glucose or glycogen for energy. This fat irritates the liver, resulting in cirrhosis, a process of swelling, scarring, and shriveling as the disease progresses.

National Council on Alcoholism and Drug Dependence
(212) 206-6770

National Institute on Alcoholism and Drug Abuse
(800) 662-4357
(301) 443-4373

Rational Recovery
(916) 621-4374

Secular Organizations for Sobriety (SOS)
(716) 834-2922

AGGRESSION

Some people are just born mean. These aggressive types tend to be angrier, noisier, pushier, and generally more hostile than their peace-loving and calmer colleagues. While some people may try to attribute these personality traits to upbringing or other environmental causes, evidence suggests that biology is to blame. In fact, in the 1970s researchers actually established a link between low levels of serotonin in the brain and aggressive behavior in animals and humans.

In studies on laboratory monkeys, those with low levels of serotonin metabolites in their blood (evidence of low levels of serotonin activity) tended to be angrier and more aggressive than the animals with normal levels of serotonin byproducts. When given drugs to boost the serotonin activity in their brains, the aggressive monkeys calmed down. Other studies showed similar behavior in rats, which became extremely aggressive when tryptophan was removed from their diet (remember, tryptophan is converted into 5-HTP and then into serotonin in the body). Peace was restored among the angry rats when the tryptophan was added to the diet.

This link between serotonin and aggression or violence appears to hold for humans as well. In 1979, a psychiatrist looked at the levels of serotonin byproducts in the blood of Navy enlisted men. He found that those men who had low levels of serotonin byproducts in their blood often had a history of aggression. Similar studies found low serotonin levels in Marines who had been discharged for excessive violence, in children who tortured animals, and in people who became violent after drinking.

These studies underscore the importance of serotonin in inhibiting violent impulses. While many people think of inhibitions as restrictive and restraining, in truth humans need some measure of inhibition or impulse control to avoid getting into trouble. Social stability requires social restraint. As individuals and as a society, our very survival would be threatened if we were impulsively to eat, drink, fight, have sex, gamble, take risks, and otherwise act without any concern for the consequences of our actions.

Although normal impulse control is taught by parents and other caregivers during the process of socialization, problems with impulse control may have their roots in physiology rather than psychology. Abnormal impulse control resulting in aggression and other antisocial behavior often involves a biological problem related to serotonin activity; it does not always reflect a social or emotional problem based on "not learning how to behave."

The nutritional supplement 5-HTP can be helpful in moderating aggression. It has been established that people with a history of violence against others and against the self (those who attempt suicide or self-mutilation) often suffer from low serotonin levels in the brain. Research has shown that these people tend to improve and show fewer signs of aggression and violence when they receive supplemental tryptophan 5-HTP.

If you tend to behave aggressively in your interactions with others (or you feel out of control when you become angry), you might want to discuss taking supplemental 5-HTP with your physician to see if it can soothe your mood and make you feel less hostile. (For more information on using 5-HTP, see Chapter 6, "The Safe and Effective Use of 5-HTP.")

CALL FOR HELP

International Society for Research on Aggression
Institute for Social Research
University of Michigan
426 Thompson Street
Ann Arbor, MI 48106-1248
(313) 764-8385

ANXIETY

Anxiety isn't all in your head. It is also in your pounding heart, your shallow breath, your dry mouth, your trembling hands, and your sweat-drenched brow. This physical state of high alert is accompanied by a mental state of terror, not at a specific danger but as an expression of generalized and undefined fear. Sometimes the symptoms are so severe that people having an anxiety attack end up in the hospital emergency room, convinced they are having a heart attack.

While we all feel anxious from time to time, uncontrolled anxiety or panic attacks can be debilitating and terrifying experiences, lasting from a few minutes to several hours or days. In some cases the episodes become chronic and ongoing, interfering with a person's ability to live a happy and productive life.

There is considerable debate about the exact causes of chronic anxiety attacks, but many experts suspect that the problem reflects an imbalance between the neurotransmitters serotonin and norepinephrine. Norepinephrine is a neurotransmitter that is part of the body's fight-or-flight stress response. It surges through the body and provides a jolt of get-up-and-go that can cause a person to feel alert in times of stress or crisis. Serotonin, on the other hand, offsets or dampens that state of high alert once the crisis has passed. Problems arise—and panic attacks may result—when the body produces too much norepinephrine and too little serotonin. When this is the case, the on switch triggering the crisis response works well, but the off switch ending the crisis response is stalled.

People who are prone to anxiety also tend to suffer from depression. The link between the two mood disorders is not completely understood, but long-term anxiety may lead to depression by producing a physical and emotional state of exhaustion. Or both disorders could be independently linked to an imbalance in the levels of neurotransmitters in the brain.

A number of medications and psychological treatments can be helpful in managing anxiety. In particular, serotonin-active drugs (such as SSRIs) tend to be quite effective (perhaps because one of the suspected roles of serotonin is to reduce anxiety). While these drugs can be effective, so can the natural supplement 5-HTP, which tends to cause fewer side effects.

For example, a 1985 study from the *Journal of Affective Disorders* found a significant reduction in anxiety (as measured by three different scales) in ten patients with anxiety disorders who were given supplemental 5-HTP. In another study of twenty people with panic disorder, many experienced a feeling of "relief" after taking 5-HTP.

If you occasionally feel anxious or sometimes suffer from panic disorder (and you are not already taking any medications that alter your serotonin levels), you and your doctor might consider the use of 5-HTP to minimize the frequency or intensity of your feelings of anxiety. (For more information on using 5-HTP, see Chapter 6, "The Safe and Effective Use of 5-HTP.")

CALL FOR HELP

Anxiety Disorders Association of America
6000 Executive Boulevard, Suite 513
Rockville, MD 20852
(301) 231-9350

Council on Anxiety Disorders
P.O. Box 17011
Winston-Salem, NC 27116
(910) 722-7760

National Mental Health Association
1021 Prince Street
Alexandria, VA 22314
(703) 684-7722

CARDIOVASCULAR DISEASE

In a healthy adult, the heart beats about 10,000 times a day, pumping the equivalent of more than 4,000 gallons of blood through a complex, 12,400-mile network of arteries, veins, and blood vessels. That's an impressive accomplishment, one that underscores the importance of maintaining a well-tuned heart and cardiovascular system.

You are no doubt aware of the importance of diet and exercise in preventing heart disease, but you may not know that the neurotransmitter serotonin, found in the platelets (the blood cells that help to close wounds and promote healing), plays a complex but critical role in regulating blood flow to the brain, heart, and gastrointestinal tract. In addition, serotonin regulates the flexibility of the blood vessels, causing them to expand (acting as a vasodilator) or to contract (acting as a vaso-constrictor).

Because serotonin has such an important effect on blood pressure and blood flow, many experts suspect that abnormal seroto-nin levels may contribute to several types of cardiovascular disease. These serotonin-dependent conditions include hypertension (or high blood pressure), peripheral vascular disease (or circulatory problems in the ex-tremities, such as the hands and feet), and Raynaud's disease (a condition in which the fingers or toes become numb and discolored when exposed to cold).

Studies indicate that the amino acid tryp-tophan can be helpful in the treatment of these cardiovascular problems because it helps to relax the muscles in the vessel walls. In fact, one 1982 study found that tryptophan was able to lower the expected rate of deaths from heart attacks by 15 percent. Basically, the tryptophan worked by soothing the heart muscle and lowering the chances that the heart would spasm and go into fibrillation or uncontrolled fluttering.

As you know, tryptophan is no longer available without a doctor's prescription. You can talk to your doctor about using over-the-counter 5-HTP or tryptophan supplements (by prescription). Unlike other conditions in which you strive to get as much 5-HTP into the brain as possible, when 5-HTP is used to help manage cardiovascular illness the goal is to keep a significant portion of it outside the brain. To encourage the amount of 5-HTP outside the brain, take a dose of 5-HTP at the same time you eat a protein-rich meal to block the passage of 5-HTP to the brain. In most cases, try to consume 5-HTP between meals to maximize absorption by the brain. (For more information on using 5-HTP, see Chapter 6, "The Safe and Effective Use of 5-HTP.")

CALL FOR HELP

American Heart Association
7272 Greenville Avenue
Dallas, TX 75231
(214) 373-6300

International Atherosclerosis Society
6550 Fannin, No. 1423
Houston, TX 77030
(713) 790-4226

Mended Hearts
7272 Greenville Avenue
Dallas, TX 75231-4966
(214) 706-1442

National Heart, Lung and Blood Institute
Information Center
National Institutes of Health
P.O. Box 30105
Bethesda, MD 20824-0105
(301) 251-1222

National Heart Savers Association
9140 West Dodge Road
Omaha, NE 68114
(402) 398-1993

National Hypertension Association
324 East 30 Street
New York, NY 10016
(212) 889-3557

DEMENTIA AND ALZHEIMER'S DISEASE

One of the advantages of growing older is that we accumulate the wisdom and precious memories of a lifetime. Unfortunately, Alzheimer's disease and dementia can rob us of this knowledge, which is part of what makes us who we are.

At least four million Americans suffer from Alzheimer's disease, yet medical researchers do not yet know what causes it. In some cases, a genetic problem or abnormality has been identified, but experts believe that most of the time the problem is caused by environmental factors, such as viruses or toxic exposures.

The disease is characterized by a series of symptoms, which usually become progressively worse over time. These symptoms include:

- memory loss (an impaired ability to learn new information or to recall previously learned information)
- language disturbance (the inability to recall words)
- impaired motor function
- problems recognizing or identifying common objects
- impaired "executive" functioning (planning, organizing, sequencing, and abstracting skills)

These problems are symptomatic of dementia and Alzheimer's if they are not caused by another known problem of the central nervous system, such as Parkinson's disease, a brain tumor, or vascular disease in the brain. In addition, people with Alzheimer's develop mood and behavior changes; they may become anxious or depressed, or sometimes aggressive and violent. In many cases, these emotional and behavioral changes can be more difficult for other family members to accept than the deterioration of mental capacity.

It appears that the symptoms of Alzheimer's result from the loss of cells in several key areas of the brain. This, in turn, reduces the levels of acetylcholine, the neurotransmitter largely responsible for memory. In addition to the chemical changes, the brain of an Alzheimer's patient is physically changed—it develops tangles or growths in the tissue, as well as abnormal plaques or deposits.

Changes in serotonin activity may have an influence on some of the mood changes associated with Alzheimer's disease. In fact, researchers who have conducted postmortem examinations of the brains of Alzheimer's patients found evidence of serious damage to the serotonin system. This finding was not surprising, since serotonin does have an effect on memory, mood, aggression, and impulse control.

Drugs designed to alter serotonin levels, such as SSRIs, have been effective in controlling or minimizing some of the mood and behavior changes of many Alzheimer's patients. In some cases, the ability to control the emotional upheavals can be enough to enable the family to care for the Alzheimer's patient at home a bit longer before requiring institutional care.

A study done in 1977 found that there was an improvement in the levels of the metabolites of serotonin (indicating a more active serotonin system) after the participants received 5-HTP. Another study done of twenty-four patients with senile dementia in 1981 determined that an increase in tryptophan absorption was necessary for an improvement in mental functioning.

If someone you know with Alzheimer's disease or dementia suffers from depression, anxiety, or uncharacteristic aggression that may be attributed to low serotonin function, consider having him or her take a 5-HTP supplement every day (if the person's primary physician agrees to the treatment). The nutrition supplement will not reverse the condition, but it may be able to stall or delay some of the difficult emotional changes that often accompany Alzheimer's disease and dementia.

CALL FOR HELP

Alzheimer's Disease and Related Disorders Association
919 North Michigan Avenue, Suite 1000
Chicago, IL 60611
(312) 335-8700
(800) 272-3900

Alzheimer's Disease Society
2 West 45 Street, Room 1703
New York, NY 10036
(212) 719-4744

American Journal of Alzheimer's Care and Related Disorders
470 Boston Post Road
Weston, MA 02193
(617) 899-2702

Association for Alzheimer's and Related Diseases
70 East Lake Street, Suite 600
Chicago, IL 60601-5997
(800) 572-6037
(800) 621-0379

FIBROMYALGIA

Until recently, people suffering from fibromyalgia got no respect. They went from doctor to doctor seeking help, only to be told their problems were all in their heads. For the person with the condition, the chronic muscle and joint pain, sleep disturbances, depression, anxiety, headaches, and bowel problems were all too real. Fortunately, in recent years most doctors have become better educated about the realities of fibromyalgia and better able to help their patients cope with the disease.

Fibromyalgia is often discussed along with chronic fatigue syndrome, a condition characterized by prolonged, debilitating exhaustion. Together, fibromyalgia and chronic fatigue syndrome afflict between three and six million Americans, mostly women.

5-HTP has been proved very effective at lessening the symptoms of fibromyalgia. Research conducted in Florence, Italy, in 1996 found that serotonin was very helpful in treating both fibromyalgia and migraine headaches. (Many people who suffer from fibromyalgia also suffer from migraines.) According to the study, people taking a combination of 5-HTP and the MAO inhibitors enjoyed significant improvement.

In 1992, another study found the nutritional supplement 5-HTP to be very effective at improving symptoms of fibromyalgia, even when it is taken alone. In a three-month study of fifty patients suffering from primary fibromyalgia syndrome, half the participants experienced "good" or "fair" clinical improvement. The study took into account a range of variables, including number of tender points, anxiety, level of pain, quality of sleep, and overall fatigue.

If you suffer from fibromyalgia, talk to your doctor about taking 5-HTP to help ease the pain and refresh your mood. (For more information on using 5-HTP, see Chapter 6, "The Safe and Effective Use of 5-HTP.")

CALL FOR HELP

American Academy of Pain Management
13947 Mono Way
Sonora, CA 95370-2807
(209) 533-9744

American Pain Society
4700 West Lake Avenue
Glenview, IL 60025
(847) 375-4715

Fibromyalgia Alliance of America
P.O. Box 21990
Columbus, OH 43221-0990
(614) 457-4222

International Fatigue Syndromes Share and Prayer and Pen Pal Chain
308 Stonewall Drive
Fredericksburg, VA 22401

**National Chronic Fatigue Syndrome and
Fibromyalgia Association**
P.O. Box 18426
Kansas City, MO 64133
(816) 313-2000

INSOMNIA

The more exhausted you feel, the harder it is
to fall asleep. You may toss and turn for
hours, steadily growing more anxious and
frustrated. The clock taunts you with the
passing time. Why can't you just fall asleep?

Insomnia can involve one of three sleep
disorders: difficulty falling asleep (more than
forty-five minutes), early morning awakening,
or frequent night awakenings (six or more
times). However, you have insomnia only if
these symptoms leave you feeling sleepy and
worn down during the day.

Sooner or later almost everyone experiences insomnia. Indeed, during the course of
a year, nearly one out of every three people
suffers from the problem at least once. Short-

term insomnia (lasting a few nights to a few weeks) often results from concern or worry about a stressful situation. Long-term insomnia (lasting months or years) can be triggered by a number of problems, including an imbalance in serotonin levels.

Serotonin levels fluctuate throughout a twenty-four-hour period. Serotonin activity is highest when we are awake and tapers off to almost nothing during the dream state known as REM (rapid eye movement) sleep. These changes in serotonin levels play a protective role: When serotonin levels plummet during REM sleep we are temporarily paralyzed because serotonin is necessary for voluntary muscle movement. This drop in serotonin protects us because it leaves us unable to act out our dreams.

Not surprisingly, mood disorders are often accompanied by sleep disorders, either insomnia (sleeping too little) or hypersomnia (sleeping too much). During the night, serotonin is converted by the brain into melatonin, a hormone responsible for monitoring sleep. Together, serotonin and melatonin work as a team to adjust the sleep-wake cycle. Ideally, these chemicals keep us awake and active during the day and asleep and resting at night.

Taking supplemental 5-HTP can increase and stabilize serotonin levels in your brain, which can boost your melatonin levels and improve the quality of your sleep. Research done in 1976 showed that taking 5-HTP can have a positive effect on sleep patterns. Another study done the following year found that people described as "mildly insomniac" experienced significant improvement in their sleep after taking 100 milligrams of 5-HTP before sleep.

Researchers have found 5-HTP most effective when it is taken on an empty stomach about an hour before heading for bed. If you're having trouble falling asleep and staying asleep, talk to your doctor about taking 5-HTP in the late evening. (For more information on using 5-HTP, see Chapter 6, "The Safe and Effective Use of 5-HTP.")

HAVE A BANANA BEFORE BED

Foods containing tryptophan may be able to help you fall asleep. Before bed, try munching on a midnight snack consisting of a banana, a slice of whole-grain toast with peanut butter, or a glass of milk. Many people find that these tryptophan-rich foods can help bring on sleep.

On the other hand, foods that contain tyramines cause the brain to release norepinephrine, a stimulant. Before bed, pass on tyramine-rich foods, including caffeine, alcohol, sugar, tobacco, aged cheese, chocolate, sauerkraut, wine, bacon, ham, sausage, eggplant, potatoes, spinach, and tomatoes.

CALL FOR HELP

American Sleep Disorders Institute
1610 14 Street, NW, Suite 300
Rochester, MN 55901
(507) 287-6006

Better Sleep Council
333 Commerce Street
Alexandria, VA 22314
(703) 683-8371

National Sleep Foundation
1367 Connecticut Avenue, NW, Suite 200
Washington, DC 20036
(202) 785-2300

MIGRAINE HEADACHES

A migraine is the godfather of all headaches. In many cases, a person suffering with this type of throbbing headache cannot function: The slightest movement, noise, or light can make the pain worse. To ease the pain, the migraine sufferer may retreat to a dark, quiet room to sleep off the headache, or at least to suffer without disturbance.

The excruciating pain of a migraine can be triggered by a range of dietary and environmental factors. The most common triggers include foods containing high proportions of the amino acid tyramine (red wine, aged cheeses), foods containing nitrites (processed meats), and food containing monosodium glutamate (MSG), which is included in many convenience and prepared foods.

People who suffer from migraines often

have depression as well. In fact, one study done at Case Western Reserve University found that the risk of developing depression was more than three times higher for people with migraines than those with no history of migraines. The same study found that people with a history of major depression also had more than three times the normal risk of developing migraines.

It appears that both depression and migraine headaches have the same underlying cause—serotonin deficiency. Researchers believe that people who are prone to migraines have a flaw in the serotonin receptor designed to cause the blood vessels to constrict. Certain triggers can cause the blood vessels in the brain to expand or dilate; when the vessels fill with blood, they swell and press against the surrounding tissues, causing pain and tenderness.

The most effective drugs used in the treatment of migraines (sumatriptan and ergotamine) block specific serotonin receptors in the brain. Other SSRIs prevent migraines in some people but not others. In fact, when taking SSRIs, some people experience complete relief from migraines, and for others the drug seems to intensify the pain. Researchers don't fully understand why some people experience ecstasy and others agony, but they suspect that the difference in outcome is due to the drugs' different actions on different receptor sites in the brain.

Migraine headaches can be eased through the use of the nutritional supplement 5-HTP. A Spanish study of 124 people with migraines found significant improvement in 71 percent of the people taking 5-HTP. (They experienced just as many headaches, but they were much shorter and less intense than without 5-HTP.) The authors of the study even suggested that 5-HTP could be used on an ongoing basis to prevent migraines.

A group of Italian researchers in 1986 then stepped in and showed that 5-HTP can in fact be very effective at preventing migraines. The researchers looked at forty patients with migraines; half the patients received 40 milligrams of 5-HTP a day, and the other group received a placebo. After two months, 90 percent of the people taking 5-HTP reported fewer, shorter, and milder migraines, compared to only 16 percent of the people taking the placebo.

If you have a history of migraine headaches, 5-HTP may help avoid subsequent episodes or significantly diminish their duration or intensity. (For more information on using 5-HTP, see Chapter 6, "The Safe and Effective Use of 5-HTP.")

CALL FOR HELP

American Association for the Study of Headaches
(609) 845-0322

American Council for Headache Education (ACHE)
875 Kings Highway, Suite 200
Woodbury, NJ 08096
(800) 255-ACHE
(609) 845-0322 in New Jersey

National Headache Foundation
(800) 372-7742

WOMEN AND MIGRAINES

Seven out of ten migraine suffers are women. In most cases, the headaches begin during adolescence or early adulthood, when hormone levels tend to fluctuate. Hormones appear to be a major migraine trigger in women; many women have their migraines triggered by falling estrogen levels in the days before menstruation. Birth control pills can make migraines worse, but migraines often go away during pregnancy and after menopause.

MYOCLONUS

Myoclonus is a condition characterized by brief, involuntary muscle jerks of the body, especially the arms and legs. These outbursts may occur in a rhythmic fashion or as a single jerk. The condition is sometimes referred to as "restless leg syndrome," and it occurs most frequently at night.

It can be quite disturbing, especially the first time it happens to you. One minute you're resting peacefully, and the next your arms or legs are jerking fitfully. The outburst isn't a twitch or a seizure but something in between.

Research indicates that myoclonus may be associated with low levels of serotonin in the brain. In fact, since 1975 researchers have repeatedly found that the amino acid 5-HTP can dramatically decrease the frequency and intensity of myoclonus.

For example, a study published in *The Lancet* in 1975 found that 5-HTP taken with carbidopa elevates brain levels of serotonin and diminishes the frequency of myoclonic symptoms. (See Chapter 1, "Keeping the Balance," for a description of carbidopa and other "enhancers" for 5-HTP.)

If you suffer from myoclonus, talk to your doctor about taking 5-HTP to diminish the frequency and intensity of your jerking seizures. (For more information on using 5-HTP, see Chapter 6, "The Safe and Effective Use of 5-HTP.")

CALL FOR HELP

Myoclonus Families United
1553 East 35 Street
Brooklyn, NY 11234
(718) 252-2133

PARKINSON'S DISEASE

Parkinson's is a paradoxical disease: When someone suffers from Parkinson's disease, some of the muscles become rigid and others contract involuntarily. People with Parkinson's disease may stoop, shuffle, and present a void, masklike, expressionless face while at the same time suffering from an incessant tremor in the hand. They can't move and they can't hold still.

Parkinson's disease involves a failure of the body's internal communication system. When we are healthy, we take our bodies for granted, but every move we make, from kicking a ball to writing our name, requires thousands of coordinated communications between the brain and the muscles, tendons, and bones. When these systems work well together, we think nothing of it, but when some part of the network breaks down, the effect can be devastating, as is the case with Parkinson's disease.

The disease, which afflicts more than one million Americans, involves damage to the middle section of the brain known as the substantia nigra, named for its blackish color. This midbrain area is the main supplier of dopamine, the neurotransmitter that allows communication about movement between various parts of the body. When these cells die off and the dopamine supply dwindles, the nerve signals cross and muscle action goes haywire.

Parkinson's is a degenerative disease that usually first shows up when patients are in their fifties and sixties. There is no known cure for the disease, but the symptoms can be controlled through medication and through the use of 5-HTP. Early treatment can help to slow the progress of the disease.

The cause of Parkinson's disease is unknown, though some experts suspect that a virus, malnutrition, or chemical exposure could be involved. Supporting evidence for the virus-trigger theory is that many people who survived the encephalitis epidemics between 1919 and 1926 (caused by a virus) developed Parkinson's years later. The toxin-trigger theory was bolstered by evidence of an outbreak of a Parkinson's-like disorder among drug addicts in San Francisco in the early 1980s.

The symptoms of Parkinson's disease are known to result from neurotransmitter imbalances following the loss of nerve cells that produce dopamine. This imbalance can be partially remedied through drug treatment.

Studies show that people with Parkinson's disease are more prone to depression than people with other progressive and disabling disease. This finding suggests that changes in the balance of dopamine and serotonin may contribute to the depression.

Researchers have evaluated the levels of serotonin and related substances in the cerebrospinal fluid of patients with Parkinson's disease. They found low levels of 5-HTP, compared to the controls who did not have Parkinson's.

If you or someone you love suffers from Parkinson's disease and you are not taking other drugs that affect the neurotransmitters, talk to your doctor about taking supplemental 5-HTP in order to increase serotonin activity in the brain. In this case, 5-HTP should *not* be used in place of other treatments to ease symptoms. (For more information on using 5-HTP, see Chapter 6, "The Safe and Effective Use of 5-HTP.")

CALL FOR HELP

American Parkinson Disease Association
1250 Hyland Boulevard
Staten Island, NY 10305
(718) 981-8001
(800) 223-2732

National Parkinson Foundation
1501 Northwest 9 Avenue
Miami, FL 33136
(800) 327-4545

WHEN IT ISN'T PARKINSON'S DISEASE

Some people develop symptoms of Parkinson's disease that prove actually to be side effects of medications. This is called Parkinson's syndrome rather than Parkinson's disease, and the symptoms usually disappear when the drugs are discontinued. If you suspect you have Parkinson's syndrome, review your use of all prescription and nonprescription drugs and discuss the issue with your doctor.

Parkinson's Disease Foundation
William Black Medical Research Building
Columbia-Presbyterian Medical Center
650 West 168 Street
New York, NY 10032
(212) 923-4700

Parkinson Support Groups of America
11376 Cherry Hill Road, No. 204
Beltsville, MD 20705
(301) 937-1545

United Parkinson Foundation
833 West Washington Boulevard
Chicago, IL 60607
(312) 733-1893

SEASONAL AFFECTIVE DISORDER

Your moods may change from day to day, but if you come down with the "winter blues" and feel down throughout the winter months, you may be suffering from seasonal affective disorder (SAD). People who suffer from SAD may experience depression, fatigue, overeating, and oversleeping from late fall when the days grow shorter to spring when the sun comes out again.

SAD is caused by reduced exposure to sunlight. While the exact mechanism is not understood, people who come down with the winter blues may have an internal clock that does not adjust very well to changes in light. Or the change in light exposure may affect melatonin production, which in turn affects the sleep cycle and overall mood.

SAD is a surprisingly common problem. Based on surveys, about half of all people in the northern U.S. feel worse in the winter than during other seasons, and an estimated one in four Americans has at least mild SAD.

In studies and surveys, people with SAD report sleeping an average of 2.5 hours more per night in the winter than in summer months. People with milder winter blues sleep about 1.7 hours longer.

The best treatment for SAD is increased exposure to bright light. Exercising outdoors (when weather permits), running errands on foot, and working near a window can increase exposure to light.

Increasing serotonin production by taking supplemental 5-HTP may help to ease symptoms. While studies have not been done that expressly demonstrated the link between 5-HTP and SAD, many of the symptoms of SAD involve serotonin-related problems, such as depression, overeating, and sleep disturbance. If you suffer from SAD, you might want to check with your doctor about using 5-HTP on an experimental basis to see if it improves your mood. (For more information, see Chapter 6, "The Safe and Effective Use of 5-HTP.")

CALL FOR HELP

**Depression and Related Affective Disorders
Association**
Johns Hopkins Hospital
600 North Wolfe Street
Baltimore, MD 21287
(410) 955-4647

**Depressives Anonymous: Recovering from
Depression**
329 East 62 Street
New York, NY 10021
(212) 689-2600

**Foundation for Depression and Manic
Depression**
24 East 81 Street, Suite 2B
New York, NY 10028
(212) 772-3400

National Depressive and Manic Depressive Association
730 North Franklin Street, Suite 501
Chicago, IL 60610
(312) 642-0049
(800) 826-3632

National Foundation for Depressive Illness
P.O. Box 2257
New York, NY 10116
(212) 268-4260

National Mental Health Association
1021 Prince Street
Alexandria, VA 22314
(703) 684-7722
(800) 243-2525

Part 3

USING 5-HTP

6. THE SAFE AND EFFECTIVE USE OF 5-HTP

NOW THAT YOU HAVE READ THE PREVIOUS CHAP-
ters, you know that 5-HTP can help to lift
your depressed mood, diminish cravings and
eating compulsions, ease you into a good
night's sleep, and assist in the treatment of a
number of other health problems. You also
know that 5-HTP is not only effective but also
remarkably free of the side effects often associated with drugs used to treat these problems.

If you are ready to join the thousands of
Americans who are already benefiting from

this nutritional supplement, this chapter will help you devise your own 5-HTP treatment plan. Of course, you should be aware that 5-HTP is not a miracle cure. The health problems discussed in this book are often complex and multifaceted. While 5-HTP may be an important part of your treatment plan, you should use the nutritional supplement as part of a comprehensive strategy for improved health. *You should discuss your overall treatment plan with your doctor or health professional.*

If you are currently taking prescription drugs to treat depression, anxiety, migraine headaches, eating disorders, or any other medical condition discussed in this book, do not discontinue your treatment or medication without consulting your doctor. Stopping drug treatment abruptly can put you at risk of developing serious physical and emotional symptoms, depending on the medication you are taking.

IS 5-HTP RIGHT FOR YOU?

As the previous chapters have shown, 5-HTP can work wonders for many people, but it is not safe for everyone. The nutritional supplement can cause drug interactions if taken with certain medications, and it should be avoided by people with certain medical profiles. Everyone should discuss treatment with a physician *before* using 5-HTP, especially the following individuals:

People on Certain Medications

- People who take serotonin reuptake inhibitors (SSRIs). These include:
    fluoxetine (Prozac)
    venlafaxine (Effexor)
    paroxetine (Paxil)
    sertraline (Zoloft)
    bupropion (Wellbutrin, Zyban)

- People taking other antidepressants, especially MAO inhibitors. These include:

> phenelzine (Nardil)
> tranylcypromine (Parnate)

- People taking prescription and over-the-counter weight-loss drugs
- People taking L-dopa (used in the treatment of Parkinson's disease)
- People taking drugs that can damage the liver, such as chemotherapy (as part of a cancer treatment) or powerful antibiotics (to combat severe infection)

People with Certain Medical Conditions

- Pregnant women and nursing mothers
- People with AIDS or HIV infection
- People with a predisposition to a type of heart disease known as endomyocardial fibrosis
- Alcoholics with compromised liver function
- People with cirrhosis of the liver or hepatitis
- People suffering from gastrointestinal disorders, such as ulcers, irritable bowel disease,

    Crohn's disease, or an extremely sensitive
    GI tract

- People with lupus or other autoimmune disorders

- People with severe bronchial asthma

- People with a hindgut carcinoid tumor. This rare disease is characterized by tumors of serotonin-forming cells in the gut or lungs; it is associated with extremely high levels of serotonin in the blood.

If you're intrigued by the possibilities of using 5-HTP, but you fall into one of the categories listed above, don't despair. You may be able to include 5-HTP in your treatment plan, but the key issue is that you discuss the matter with your doctor first.

MAKING 5-HTP WORK FOR YOU

If you have decided to try 5-HTP to improve your health you must learn more about how to maximize the effectiveness of the supplement. Keep in mind that research shows that

WHY PEOPLE ON SSRIS SHOULD AVOID 5-HTP

For the past few years, SSRIs (selective serotonin reuptake inhibitors) have been replacing tricyclic antidepressants as the drug of choice to treat depression in the United States. According to researchers at the Department of Emergency Medicine, University of Pittsburgh, serotonin syndrome is a severe adverse drug interaction associated with SSRIs.

In an article published in 1996 in the *Annals of Emergency Medicine*, the researchers noted that serotonin syndrome is characterized by the combination of altered mental state, problems with the autonomous nervous system (which regulates involuntary action, such as the intestines, heart, and glands) and neuromusclar abnormalities. Researchers speculate that the condition may be caused by excessive levels of 5-HTP (which, in turn, become serotonin in the brain). For this reason, people taking SSRIs should not use 5-HTP without a doctor's consent.

the dosage and usage information are the same for the treatment of all conditions. In other words, the key points listed below apply whether you're using 5-HTP to control depression, eating disorders, insomnia, or some other condition discussed in this book or known to be caused by low levels of serotonin in the brain.

Between 50 and 200 Milligrams of 5-HTP a Day Is Considered the Therapeutic Dose

Most over-the-counter 5-HTP capsules come in 50-milligram doses. Typically people can safely consume up to 200 milligrams of 5-HTP a day without adverse side effects. In the body, 100 milligrams of 5-HTP produce a rise in the blood plasma concentration of serotonin equal to the amount that would occur if a person ate about 10 bananas. This is the therapeutic dose for the medical conditions discussed in this book. Doctors occasionally recommend higher doses.

If you took tryptophan in the past, you will find that 5-HTP is about five to ten times more powerful. In other words, if you used to take 500 milligrams of L-tryptophan to treat a stubborn bout of insomnia, you would need to take only about 100 milligrams of 5-HTP to enjoy the same soothing benefit. Much higher doses of 5-HTP have been prescribed in the treatment of some disorders.

For some chronic conditions, a maintenance dose is sometimes recommended. In such cases, just 100 milligrams of 5-HTP a day is usually effective.

Take 5-HTP on an Empty Stomach

5-HTP works best if it is taken three or more hours after your last protein-containing meal or snack and a half hour before your next meal. Washing it down with any type of fruit juice can also give it a boost. (The carbohydrate helps clear the way for the serotonin-producing amino acids to enter the brain.)

Take 5-HTP and a Good Multivitamin/mineral Supplement

Vitamin B_6 helps the body convert 5-HTP into serotonin in the brain. More than twenty years ago, researchers established the link between vitamin B_6 and serotonin when they deliberately induced a state of vitamin B_6 deficiency in rats. They found that very little serotonin was produced in the rat brain when it did not have enough vitamin B_6.

Other experiments with monkeys and rats conducted in the 1990s have shown that the presence of ample amounts of vitamin B_6 (even to the point of "moderate excess") increases production of serotonin in the brain from 5-HTP by up to 60 percent.

To ensure that you're taking enough vitamin B_6, take a comprehensive multivitamin (containing at least 10 milligrams of vitamin B_6), or a B-complex vitamin (most of which contain either 25 or 50 milligrams of each of the B vitamins). You need to take the entire B complex rather than simply B_6 because the B vitamins work in harmony; taking one in isolation can lead to an imbalance in the other B vitamins.

Do Not Drink Alcohol While Taking 5-HTP

Alcohol affects the metabolism of 5-HTP. If you use 5-HTP, do not drink alcohol for at least six hours before its use. Also, alcoholics and people with cirrhosis of the liver or liver damage due to excessive drinking should not use 5-HTP.

Take Steps to Minimize Side Effects

According to a review of the scientific literature, the most common unwelcome side effect associated with the use of 5-HTP is gastrointestinal upset, including gas, nausea, diarrhea, and cramping. This GI upset happens to only a minority of users, and even then only occasionally. It usually tapers off and disappears after a few days or weeks of use.

The risk of GI upset can be minimized by starting with a low dose (25 to 50 milligrams) and increasing the dose slowly (every three to five days) to a maximum of 200 milligrams daily. If your stomach bothers you, try dividing your total daily intake of 5-HTP into two to four doses, with no more than 100 milligrams per dose. If GI upset remains a problem, try taking 5-HTP with food, but not with high-protein foods, since protein can undermine its effectiveness.

Some people feel groggy or sleepy after taking 5-HTP. If you experience this side effect, take 5-HTP only at night, when you're ready to welcome some shut-eye.

QUESTIONS AND ANSWERS ABOUT 5-HTP

How long will I have to take 5-HTP before I start to see—and feel—the results?

Amino acids begin to take effect within an hour or so, and you may feel some improvement almost immediately, depending on the symptoms you are trying to treat. For example, the sleep-enhancing benefits of 5-HTP may kick in within an hour or so, but it may take several days before you begin to feel a significant change in your moods or appetite.

To give 5-HTP a fair chance to prove itself, use the nutritional supplement for at least two weeks. If you suffer from a condition associated with ongoing serotonin deficiency, your doctor may recommend that you take 5-

HTP indefinitely on a maintenance dose (rather than at a higher, therapeutic dose).

Once I start to feel better, do I need to continue taking 5-HTP?

It depends. Once the nutritional supplement has helped to relieve the symptoms or medical condition—whether the problem was depression or insomnia—you can discuss with your doctor either quitting 5-HTP or continuing on the maintenance level 100 milligrams or less. Since many of the conditions described in this book involve chronic health problems, an ongoing low-dose regimen may be the most successful.

Of course, you can stop taking 5-HTP at any time. As with any drug, it is best gradually to taper off the dosage over several days, rather than suddenly stop.

Do I need to take 5-HTP in conjunction with other drugs to minimize adverse reactions?

No. Recent research has shown that 5-HTP is most effective when taken without enhancers. Several years ago researchers worried about a theoretical risk that 5-HTP could cause dangerously high blood levels of serotonin. For a time, drugs known as peripheral decarboxylase inhibitors (PDIs) were used along with 5-HTP to inhibit an enzyme that can convert 5-HTP to serotonin in the intestines and other organs (rather than in the brain). Theoretically, unless the enzyme is blocked by PDIs such as carbidopa or benserazide, 5-HTP would be converted to serotonin in the blood (where it can cause problems at high levels) rather than in the brain (where it can cause the health benefits outlined in this book).

Defenders of 5-HTP note, however, that scientific studies have not supported the use of PDIs with 5-HTP. 5-HTP is apparently no more effective when used with a PDI, and when taken with a PDI, people taking 5-HTP experienced more side effects. As for the risk of heart attack or organ damage, defenders point out that after twenty-five years of research, no serious health effects such as heart attacks have ever been recorded in 5-HTP studies or clinical use.

The authors of a study that looked at 5-HTP's adverse effects noted, "Researchers who reported on the results of various laboratory functions (hematologic, liver, kidney, etc.) found that 5-HTP caused no significant changes . . . oral administration of 5-HTP without carbidopa is associated with few adverse side effects." (For a discussion of the efficacy of PDIs, see Chapter 1, "Keeping the Balance.")

Do I need to test my urine levels for evidence of serotonin activity if I take 5-HTP?

No. Some people believe that they should test their urine for high levels of 5-HIAA, a metabolite of serotonin. There is no evidence to suggest that taking the dose of 5-HTP recommended in this book can elevate serotonin levels to a harmful level.

Why do I need to take 5-HTP supplements if I make a point to eat enough protein (which contains tryptophan, the amino acid that is converted to 5-HTP in the body)?

Because your body may not be able to convert the protein you eat into serotonin you can use. It's true that the average American adult consumes an estimated 90 to 100 grams of protein a day, an amount that is more than twice the Recommended Daily Allowance of 44 to 56 grams a day. This excess protein doesn't have a dramatic effect on serotonin production because the other amino acids in the protein compete with tryptophan to enter the brain. (Remember, tryptophan can cross into the brain only when there is more of it than other amino acids in the blood.) In addition, poor dietary patterns can interfere with the conversion of protein to serotonin.

However, it is worth noting that what you eat can influence the effectiveness of 5-HTP. Chapter 7, "Eat Smart: The 5-HTP–Enhancing Diet," can help you choose foods that will boost your levels of 5-HTP and allow your body to use that 5-HTP more effectively, whether or not you take any additional nutritional supplements.

Is there any kind of test I can take to find out if my body is low in tryptophan or 5-HTP?

Yes, but it isn't necessary for most people. Most individuals can go ahead and take 5-HTP without risk of serotonin overdose, provided they consume only the amounts recommended in this book.

If you are concerned about your overall amino acid profile, you can take a quantitative urinary amino acid screening test. As part of the test, you must collect all of your urine for a twenty-four-hour period. Some amino acids spill into the urine, so researchers can get a fairly good amino acid profile by analyzing the sample. The sample findings are then compared against the expected average, so that any imbalances or deficiencies can be noted.

If you want a urine screening test, discuss the matter with your doctor or a nutritionist. The tests are becoming more popular, but facilities are still not widely available. If you can't find a laboratory near you that does the testing, contact one of the following labs:

- Medabolics, 573 Hillcrest Drive, Paradise, CA 95969

- SmithKline Bio-Science Laboratories, 7600 Tyrone Avenue, Van Nuys, CA 91405

- Doctor's Data, 30 West 101 Roosevelt Road, West Chicago, IL 60185

- Riner's, 1713 Midcrest, Plano, TX 75075 (214) 422–0848

How much does 5-HTP cost?

The cost of a 10-milligram capsule can range from about 50¢ to $2, depending on the manufacturer. Because of this incredible difference in price, be sure to compare costs. When comparison shopping, make sure you compare the prices of pills of comparable strength. For example, don't compare the price of a 50-milligram capsule with the cost of a 100-milligram capsule.

Can I get my insurance company to pay for my 5-HTP as part of my treatment plan?

Probably not. Because 5-HTP is a nutritional supplement rather than a drug, it is not covered by most insurance plans. (Under some insurance plans it may be covered if it is prescribed by a doctor.) Of course, it can't hurt to ask. If your doctor is willing to do so, you may ask him or her to write a note to the insurance company explaining that the 5-HTP is part of a treatment program.

Does the U.S. Food and Drug Administration test 5-HTP to make sure that the products I buy are safe and effective?

No. The FDA doesn't monitor nutritional supplements in the same way that it does prescription and over-the-counter drugs. When it comes to drug manufacture, the FDA pays close attention to quality control and production; you can be confident that a medication contains the ingredients in the amounts stated on the product label.

The manufacture of nutritional supplements does not receive the same level of government scrutiny. Many manufacturers do, however, provide their own quality control measures. Some companies heed standards that rival those of drug manufacturers. If you want to know about how a batch of 5-HTP has been made by a particular manufacturer, write or call the company and ask for information on their quality control measures and their production process. Nutritional supplement manufacturers that take special care with their quality control should be pleased to tell you all about their procedures. The phone numbers and address of some companies that manufacture 5-HTP are listed in Chapter 9, "Where to Find 5-HTP." If you're interested in buying a product from a different manufacturer, look for the address on the product label.

I know that 5-HTP can be helpful in controlling cravings for alcohol, yet it is not recommended for alcoholics. Why?

Because advanced alcoholics may have experienced liver damage, which can make it impossible for the body properly to metabolize 5-HTP. (For the same reason, people who are intravenous drug users and those with cirrhosis of the liver, hepatitis, or parasitic infections should not use 5-HTP.)

Animal studies show that taking 5-HTP without adequate liver function can lead to serious complications. In a study on animals receiving both 5-HTP and liver toxic drugs (to simulate liver damage), the animals developed heart fibrosis, or deposits of connective tissue in the heart muscle.

If you have a history of heavy alcohol use and you want to take 5-HTP to help control alcohol cravings, ask your doctor to perform a test of your liver function. This inexpensive test will indicate whether your liver is healthy enough to metabolize 5-HTP and other nutritional supplements.

7. EAT SMART: THE 5-HTP–ENHANCING DIET

THE FOODS YOU EAT, AND WHEN YOU EAT THEM, can have a profound influence on the levels of 5-HTP and serotonin in your body. The 5-HTP–enhancing diet described in this chapter can help you maximize serotonin production in your brain, whether or not you take 5-HTP as a nutritional supplement.

As you know, the amino acid tryptophan is used to produce serotonin in the brain and throughout the body. Tryptophan is an essential amino acid, meaning that the body needs it to be healthy, but it cannot synthesize it from other substances in the diet. Fortunately, tryptophan is found in abundance in all high-protein foods, including dairy products, eggs, meat, and fish. (Vegetarians need not fear; tryptophan is also found in seeds, nuts, and a number of vegetables.)

Foods containing tryptophan contain a number of other amino acids. When your body digests the foods you eat, the amino acids in those foods enter the bloodstream and circulate throughout the body. The body then uses the amino acids, including tryptophan, to create the body's own proteins, as well as other molecules such as serotonin.

It seems reasonable to assume that to raise serotonin levels, you should eat high-protein foods because they contain high levels of tryptophan. Feeling down? Have a cheeseburger and a shake. About to get a crashing migraine headache? Have a big plate of scrambled eggs and sausage. While this approach might seem logical, the opposite is true: High-protein meals can actually impair serotonin production. Instead, you need to munch on well-timed high-carbohydrate snacks and meals to maximize the levels of tryptophan in the brain.

THE CARBOHYDRATE CONNECTION

Researchers now know that the foods you eat can have a significant impact on your mood and mind-set, but before 1972 most researchers dismissed claims about the mood-altering effects of foods (except, of course, the effects of caffeine and alcohol). They knew that the brain was protected by the blood-brain barrier, which filters many substances from the bloodstream and slows the passage of large molecules into the brain. Oxygen and sugar can slip past and enter the brain without delay, but amino acids (such as tryptophan) are so big that they must wait with the other large molecules to pass slowly through a narrow passage into the brain. According to the state-of-the-art science of the early 1970s, food could not influence mood because the blood-brain barrier served as such a powerful protective mechanism. Tryptophan entered the brain at a fixed rate of speed, and diet played

no role in its availability—or so the researchers assumed.

This dietary paradigm abruptly changed in
1972 when Dr. John Fernstrom and Dr. Rich-
ard Wurtman of the Massachusetts Institute
of Technology published their landmark
study on carbohydrates and brain serotonin
in the journal *Science*. The researchers
showed that the protein and carbohydrate
content of a meal or snack has a significant
impact of the production of serotonin.

Since then, researchers have gained a much
greater understanding of the importance of
diet in the formation of neurotransmitters.
Animal studies have shown that adding small
amounts of protein to a carbohydrate food can
render the carbohydrate powerless to raise serotonin levels in the brain. In fact, one study
on rats found that adding just 5 percent protein to a carbohydrate snack is enough to offset the meal's ability to stimulate serotonin
activity.

Carbohydrates, on the other hand, clear the
way for tryptophan to cross the blood-brain
barrier. The carbohydrates cause the pancreas

to release insulin (which lowers the amount of sugar in the bloodstream). The insulin also forces the amino acids in the bloodstream (except for tryptophan) to make their way into the body's tissues to build protein. During this process, the concentration of tryptophan in the blood rises because the other amino acids clear out. Since there are fewer amino acids waiting to cross the blood-brain barrier, the tryptophan is able to enter the brain at higher levels. In effect, the carbohydrates have knocked out the competition, giving tryptophan easier access to the brain. The bottom line: It is carbohydrate consumption, not protein consumption, that determines how much tryptophan can enter the brain.

Quite a few animal studies have shown that high-carbohydrate meals increase levels of tryptophan and serotonin levels in the brain. Studies with humans have looked at moods and energy levels after people eat both protein and carbohydrate meals. In general, people (especially those with serotonin deficiency) report a lift in mood after eating carbohydrates.

WHAT TO EAT

To boost levels of tryptophan, 5-HTP, and serotonin in the brain, choose high-
carbohydrate foods such as whole-grain
breads, cereals, pasta, potatoes, and fruits.
These foods can provide a long-lasting mood
and energy boost. High-fat or high-sugar carbohydrates offer the same serotonin-boosting
benefits (as well as momentary pleasure), but
they are often followed by a rapid return of
appetite and they are nutritionally inferior to
low-fat, low-sugar alternatives.

TIMING IS EVERYTHING

For maximum benefit, you not only must eat
high-carbohydrate foods, you must eat them
at the appropriate times. A number of experiments done with laboratory animals have determined how to time the meals to increase
brain serotonin levels.

Ideally, to boost tryptophan, 5-HTP, and serotonin levels, avoid protein in the morning.

Do eat breakfast, but be sure that your breakfast consists of carbohydrates but little or no protein. Using this approach, there should be a significant increase in brain serotonin levels two to three hours after eating.

Research has shown that if you consumed mostly protein at breakfast, you would experience no increase in serotonin levels. Your brain serotonin levels would also stay flat if you ate a combination of carbohydrates and proteins. In other words, if your first meal of the day is eggs, bacon, and toast, this meal contains too much protein to increase serotonin production, even though you might experience the mild, momentary mood lift that usually follows every meal.

All the studies done to date indicate that you need to eat your high-carbohydrate meal or snack on an empty stomach in order to achieve a noticeable boost in serotonin activity in the brain. In laboratory rats, an interval of three hours seems to be the minimum needed to clear the protein from an earlier meal. (It may be somewhat longer—perhaps four hours—for human beings, because we have a slower metabolic rate than rats.) If you eat a high-carbohydrate meal or snack relatively soon after a protein or a mixed protein-carbohydrate meal, it will do nothing to boost serotonin levels. To enjoy the serotonin-enhancing benefits of carbohydrates, you need to wait about three or four hours after eating protein.

Of course, you should not entirely eliminate protein from your daily diet. Instead, consume one or two ounces of protein at lunch and most of the protein in your diet for dinner, the final meal of the day. In terms of controlling serotonin activity during the day, breakfast is the most important meal of the day.

Don't worry about skimping on protein. The average American consumes more than twice as much protein as is necessary for health. Vegetables and complex carbohydrates contain small amounts of protein. For most people, as little as two ounces of animal protein (milk, meat, fish, or poultry) is plenty.

During the day, if you start to drag in the midmorning or afternoon, snack on high-carbohydrate foods. Avoid eating high-fat or high-sugar snacks; instead, opt for complex carbohydrates, which tend to provide better nutrition and can improve overall health. The following categories can help you plan your meal and snack selections.

Good Choices for Breakfast: No Protein

Dry cereal with skim milk
Oatmeal, cream of wheat, or Wheatena
Whole-grain toast
Waffles or pancakes
Mixed fruit
Fruit juice
Muffin with preserves

FOODS TO AVOID: BACON, SAUSAGE, EGGS, CHEESE, AND OTHER HIGH-PROTEIN FOODS

Good Choices for Lunch: One or Two Ounces of Protein

Pasta or pasta salad with vegetables (no meat)

Caesar salad
French bread pizza
Vegetable or bean soup
Vegetables with rice
Vegetable sandwich on whole-wheat bread
or pita

FOODS TO AVOID: LARGE PORTIONS OF MEAT,
POULTRY, FISH, OR DAIRY

*Good Choices for Dinner: Two or Three
Ounces of Protein*

Meat, fish, poultry, or tofu
Vegetables
Starches

FOODS TO AVOID: HIGH-FAT AND HIGH-SUGAR
FOODS, WHICH CAN INCREASE APPETITE AND HAVE
NO ROLE IN A WELL-BALANCED DIET

Good Choices for Snacks

Fruit
Graham crackers

Pretzels

Baked potato chips

FOODS TO AVOID: HIGH-PROTEIN, HIGH-FAT, AND
HIGH-SUGAR SNACKS

You may find it helpful to keep a food journal as you experiment with the foods you eat. In a small notebook record what you eat, the time you eat it, and your mood and energy level at the time of your meal or snack. Try to make a few notes to yourself during the day to assess your physical and mental state as it fluctuates. For example, you might set up a rating system of 1 to 10 or −5 to +5. Using such a system, you could rate your mood and energy with a numerical score, which is easily compared, rather than with words, which can be harder to interpret. The food journal should be written for your own benefit, so that you can monitor how your eating patterns affect your body and mind. Don't create such an elaborate system that it will be difficult to follow because you'll be less likely to stick with it.

By paying special attention to the foods you eat and how you feel after eating them, you can discover for yourself the physical impact of eating—or avoiding—protein early in the day. Over the course of several weeks, you can fine-tune and further customize your diet so that you can boost your levels of 5-HTP and serotonin throughout the day.

NUTRITION FOR OPTIMAL HEALTH

While the 5-HTP–enhancing diet described in this chapter can help boost your serotonin levels, your overall health depends on eating a well-balanced diet. We all have different nutritional needs and food preferences, but we must work to structure a diet plan that includes both the foods we *should* eat and the foods we *want* to eat.

Four types of nutrients—carbohydrates, proteins, fats, and vitamins and minerals—work together to nourish our bodies and provide the raw materials necessary for all of our bodily processes.

- **Carbohydrates** are the body's major source
  of energy. There are two types: simple carbohydrates (sugars), which are quickly converted to blood sugar, and complex
  carbohydrates (starches), which are metabolized more slowly and provide a more
  gradual supply of energy. Complex carbohydrates take longer to burn than simple carbohydrates so they can help ward off
  between-meal hunger. Generally speaking,
  between 60 and 70 percent of the calories
  you consume each day should be carbohydrates, especially complex carbohydrates,
  such as whole-grain breads, legumes, cereals, pasta, potatoes, and other vegetables.
  When it comes to eating simple carbohydrates, try to stick to fruits, which offer vitamins and minerals in addition to sugar,
  rather than refined sugar, honey, and corn
  syrup. Remember that sugar is sugar,
  whether it goes by the name sucrose, fruc-
  tose, or maltose, and one is not better or
  worse for you than another.

  Daily goal: Six to eleven servings, including three to five servings of vegetables and

two to four servings of fruits. A serving is considered one-half cup or one slice.

- **Proteins** consist of chains of amino acids, including tryptophan. Strive to eat about 12 percent of your total calories from protein. However, as discussed earlier, avoid eating that protein early in the day. Instead, reserve most of the protein for dinner. Complete proteins (those with complete amino acids) are found in animal and plant products such as meat, fish, poultry, and dairy products.

  Daily goal: Four or five ounces a day.

- **Fats** are essential to human health. They are needed for growth, hormone production, and other essential body processes. They also carry and store fat-soluble vitamins (vitamins A, D, E, and K). And, of course, fats can make foods more palatable by adding flavor and texture.

  Daily goal: No more than 30 percent of calories from fat. (Many health authorities recommend less for optimal health.)

THE ROLE OF FATS IN A BALANCED DIET

When planning an eating strategy, many people become confused about the role of dietary fat. While fat itself does not have a negative impact on the ability of your diet to increase 5-HTP, too much fat can cause a number of health problems. In fact, experts estimate that high-fat diets contribute to at least 300,000 deaths a year. Dietary fat has been linked to atherosclerosis and heart disease, elevated blood cholesterol, high blood pressure, diabetes, arthritis, multiple sclerosis, several types of cancer, and, of course, obesity.

The typical American consumes about 40 percent of calories from fat, despite warnings that fat intake should be limited to 30 percent of calories or lower. That means about 60 to 80 grams of fat for a 1,800- to 2,400-calorie daily diet. (One gram of fat has nine calories; one gram of protein or carbohydrate has four calories.) The body needs only about 10 percent of calories from fat (about 20 grams a day) to perform its necessary functions.

In addition to watching total fat, you must keep an eye out for the type of fat you are consuming. Dietary fats consist of combinations of three types of fatty acids—saturated, polyunsaturated, and monounsaturated:

- Saturated fats tend to be hard at room temperature. Examples: Butter, cheese, chocolate, coconut oil, egg yolk, lard, meat, palm oil, vegetable shortening.

- Polyunsaturated fats tend to be liquid at room temperature. Examples: Corn, cottonseed, fish, safflower, soybean, and sunflower oils.

- Monounsaturated fats fall in between. Examples: Avocado, canola, cashew, olive, and peanut oils.

Saturated fats should be avoided as much as possible. These fats raise the level of cholesterol in the blood, which increases the risk of heart disease. In addition, saturated fats (which often come from animals) tend to contain large amounts of cholesterol. You should worry less about differentiating between mono- and polyunsaturated fats and instead focus your attention on limiting your overall fat intake, paying special care to trim the saturated fat.

Also beware of transfatty acids, which are formed when liquid oils are converted to solid fat to make margarine and vegetable shortening. In an attempt to respond to health concerns about saturated fats, food manufacturers have created transfats by bubbling hydrogen through vegetable oil in a process known as hydrogenation. The resulting partially hydrogenated vegetable oils form a semi-isolid spread (like margarine), but they contain minimal amounts of saturated fat. Although billed as heart-smart alternatives to butter because they contain little saturated fat and no cholesterol (since they come from a vegetable rather than an animal), research shows that these transfats may be as hazardous to your health and heart as old-fashioned saturated fats. One study has found that cooking with margarine (instead of liquid oil) increases the risk of heart disease by nearly 90 percent. Other studies have found that women who eat high levels of transfatty acids are at greater risk of developing breast cancer and that men who eat them are more susceptible to prostate cancer.

Is Olestra, the so-called fake fat, a better alternative? Absolutely not. Olestra is a fat substitute used in several types of snack foods, such as potato chips and corn chips. Olestra looks, tastes, and acts like real fat, but the human digestive system cannot break it down, so it passes through the body without being absorbed or adding to the tally of total calories for the day. However, Olestra does not make its way through the body unnoticed. During the journey through the digestive system, it steals from the body the fat-soluble vitamins, as well as carotenoids, important antioxidants.

You don't have to overindulge to suffer from Olestra's negative side effects. One study found that as few as six Olestra prepared potato chips (about 3 grams) caused a 20 percent drop in levels of beta-carotene and a 38 percent drop in lycopene, another carotenoid. It can also create unpleasant side effects, including anal leakage, diarrhea, intestinal cramping, and flatulence.

The bottom line: Don't look for dietary shortcuts. To protect your health, limit your fat intake to no more than 30 percent of calories from fat, with no more than 10 percent from saturated fat. Many experts recommend less, if possible.

*

A WORD ABOUT FIBER

Although it is not a nutrient, fiber is a necessary part of a well-balanced diet. Studies show that people who eat high-fiber diets have a lower risk of developing heart disease, high cholesterol, obesity, certain cancers, gallbladder disease, diverticulosis, and chronic disease of the colon.

Dietary fiber consists of complex carbohydrates and natural polymers (such as lignin), which give structure and shape to plants. There are two types of fiber—soluble and insoluble—both of which are found in fruits, vegetables, legumes, and whole grains. If you eat the high-carbohydrate diet recommended to enhance levels of 5-HTP, you should consume fiber in the vegetables, fruits, and grains included in your diet.

Soluble fiber dissolves in the digestive tract, forming a gel-like material that helps lower cholesterol levels and traps carcinogens and eliminates them from the body. Foods high in soluble fiber include oats, kidney beans, citrus fruits, apples, and potatoes.

Insoluble fiber, as the name implies, does not break down as it moves through the digestive system. This type of fiber provides the stools with the soft bulk required to absorb body waste; it also helps the intestines work smoothly and speeds the movement of the stools through the intestines. Wheat bran and whole grains, as well as the skins of many fruits and vegetables, are rich sources of this type of fiber.

Current guidelines recommend that the average adult consume at least 25 grams of fiber daily by eating a diet rich in fruits, vegetables, and whole grains. A 1996 study published in

The Journal of the American Medical Association found that men who ate more than 25 grams of fiber per day had a 36 percent lower risk of developing heart disease than those who consumed fewer than 15 grams. The study found that every 10 grams of fiber added to the diet lowered the risk of heart attack by 19 percent.

Increase your dietary fiber a little at a time, over a period of several weeks. Too much fiber at once can cause intestinal bloating, gas, and cramps. Be sure to increase your fluid intake when you increase fiber, to keep your stools soft and to avoid constipation. In general, the less processed or refined a food is, the more fiber it contains.

You can boost your fiber intake by eating the skins of potatoes, apples, and other fruits and vegetables with edible skins (after washing them thoroughly, of course.) Also opt for brown rice instead of white and whole-wheat flour instead of white. When cooking, stir-fry or steam vegetables to minimize breakdown of fiber. And add wheat bran to hot or cold cereals, sprinkle it in yogurt, mix it into casseroles, or substitute it for up to a half-cup of the flour in most baked goods.

HOW TO BOOST THE NUTRITIONAL BENEFITS OF YOUR FOODS

You may assume that eating right means simply choosing the right foods, but the choices you make when buying, storing, and preparing food can go a long way toward enhancing—or undermining—a food's nutritional value.

- *The whole is greater . . .* When shopping for cereals and grains, avoid products made with white flour; instead, choose foods made of whole grains. During the milling process, grains lose most of their vitamins and minerals, though some are added to "enriched" products.

- *Fresh or frozen?* In an ideal world, your fruits and vegetables would arrive on your plate just hours after leaving the field or gar-

THE HEALING POWER OF
COMPLEX CARBOHYDRATES

Eating a diet rich in vegetables, fruits, and grains can improve your overall health and increase the level of 5-HTP in your body. Study after study has shown that people who eat plenty of plant foods tend to suffer less from cardiovascular disease, cancer, and many other illnesses, compared with people who eat lots of meat and dairy products. Of course, plant foods tend to be high in vitamins, minerals, and fiber and low in fats and calories, but there seems to be more to it than that. Researchers now suspect that what gives these plant foods their added healing power is phytochemicals, or plant chemicals.

To the best of our understanding, phytochemicals work as part of a plant's antioxidant defense system, and they also help the plant survive viral attack and difficult weather. In humans, phytochemicals have no known nutritional value, and they do not add to the caloric content of food. But they do seem to have a remarkable ability to help fight cancer, prevent cell damage, and suppress malignant changes in cells when they do occur.

All plants contain a number of phytochemicals. While some have been isolated and offered for sale as nutritional supplements, it is best to get your daily dose of phytochemicals by eating a diet high in fruit and vegetables. At this point scientists do not know whether specific phytochemicals act alone to fight disease, or whether they work synergistically with other plant chemicals. So boost your 5-HTP levels and improve your overall health at the same time by eating your vegetables.

den. But in the real world, produce spends days or weeks in transit, losing vitamins and minerals each day. If you're in doubt about the freshness of the produce in your market, don't hesitate to choose frozen. The flash-freezing process used to prepare frozen foods protects all the vitamins except vitamin E. Look for products frozen in plastic pouches; the vitamins won't wash away during cooking.

- *Can the canned vegetables.* Water-soluble vitamins leach out of the vegetables and into the water that canned vegetables are packed in, robbing them of their nutritional value. Avoid canned vegetables and fruits except when absolutely necessary. For the same reason, avoid soaking vegetables for extended periods before cooking, and steam rather than boil them to preserve their vitamin content.

- *Reduce, reuse, recycle.* If you prepare produce by boiling, use as little water as possible and reuse the water for gravies, sauces, and stocks, since this water contains many of the vitamins (as well as the flavors) of the foods cooked in it. In the morning, also drink the milk at the bottom of the cereal bowl, since this runoff contains many of the vitamins added to fortified cereals.

- *The colder, the better.* Set the temperature of your freezer at 0° F or less. At higher temperatures, foods begin to thaw, and then they lose some of their vitamins.

- *Don't let the sun shine.* To protect the riboflavin content, store milk and bread away from strong light. Avoid milk in clear glass bottles for this reason.

- *Less really is more.* With the exception of meat and poultry, which need to be thoroughly cooked, use the minimum cooking time necessary. To preserve vitamin content, high temperatures over a short period of time beat low temperatures over a longer period of time.

- *Bigger is better.* Vegetables lose less vitamin content if they are cooked whole rather than in pieces. To preserve vitamin content, cook first, then cut.

8. ANOTHER REASON TO EXERCISE: WORK OUT TO BOOST YOUR 5-HTP LEVELS

YOU ALREADY KNOW THAT EXERCISE IS GOOD for you. It can improve your physical and emotional health, reduce your risk of serious illness, rev up your sex life, and make you leaner and stronger. But exercise offers another relatively unknown benefit: It can raise levels of 5-HTP and serotonin in the brain.

Most people give endorphins all the credit for the mood-enhancing benefits of exercise, but in reality, endorphins get more credit than they deserve. Endorphins are the "feel good" chemicals released by the nerves supplying the muscles during physical exertion. These chemicals can't be responsible for the boost in mood that follows a good workout for several reasons. For one thing, most of us don't work nearly hard enough to enjoy a significant endorphin rush. You would have to run a marathon or bike one hundred miles to reach the level of exertion required to trigger a real endorphin response. In addition, the endorphins that are released do not cross the blood-brain barrier, so they cannot affect our moods.

If not endorphins, then what causes the boost in mood following exercise? The credit should go to the neurotransmitters serotonin and norepinephrine (with some small credit given to the brain endorphins). Laboratory studies have shown that brain serotonin levels doubled in animals that exercised on a treadmill for ninety minutes. Other studies have shown that people who exercise feel upbeat, even when they have been given drugs that block the effect of their endorphins.

Serotonin activity may help to explain why exercise is such an efficient antidepressant. A number of studies have shown that people who exercise regularly tend to be depressed less often than their sedentary peers of the same age and income level. In some cases, a coach can be as effective at fighting depression as a psychotherapist. In a twelve-week study at the University of Wisconsin, researchers found that working out with a personal trainer was as effective at easing moderate depression as twelve weeks of psychotherapy. When the people in the study were evaluated one year later, the exercisers were still working out and free of depression, while half of those in therapy were still in therapy or had returned with new problems.

THE BENEFITS OF EXERCISE

Most of the people who exercise regularly don't do it because they want to lose weight or stay healthy; they do it because it feels good. People who exercise regularly in moderation experience a release of tension, an easing of depression and anxiety, and even a reduction in their cravings for food and alcohol. The mood-enhancing benefits of exercise don't wear off by the time you shower and dress; exercise can improve your outlook and boost your mood for about four hours after a workout.

Exercise is also important for your overall health. Consider these benefits:

- Exercise raises levels of 5-HTP and serotonin in the brain.

- Exercise strengthens your immune system. After exercise, the number and aggressiveness of the white blood cells increase by 50 to 300 percent. It also increases the function of the body's natural killer cells, which are important in preventing cancer.

- Exercise reduces your risk of developing certain cancers, cardiovascular disease, colds and upper-respiratory tract infections, diabetes (non-insulin-dependent), high blood pressure, osteoarthritis, osteoporosis, and stroke.

- Exercise relieves anxiety, constipation, depression, low-back pain, and stress, in addition to helping you sleep at night.

- Exercise allows for the free flow of energy throughout the body.

- Exercise helps to detoxify the body and eliminate metabolic waste through sweat and accelerated respiration.

- Exercise helps you maintain and improve flexibility, stamina, and muscle strength well into old age.

- Exercise improves your mood, mental alertness, short-term memory, and reaction time.

- Exercise can help you lose weight—and keep it off.

- Exercise can help people stop drinking and using drugs; the endorphin release during exercise can provide a "natural high" that can help an addict resist temptation.

- Exercise enhances sexual desire, performance, and satisfaction.

- Exercise helps make you look years younger than your chronological age.

- Exercise helps you live longer; some studies

indicate that people who exercise regularly
live as much as two years longer than their
sedentary peers.

With so many good reasons to exercise, is
there any good reason not to?

DESIGNING A WORKOUT PLAN

"Fitness" means something different to
everyone. While it might involve breaking a
world record in the long jump for Carl Lewis,
to someone out of shape it might mean being
able to walk around the block or mow the
lawn without getting out of breath.

Although performance standards vary,
most fitness experts recognize four basic components of physical fitness:

- *Body composition:* The proportion of fat to
  bone and muscle.

- *Aerobic fitness or cardiorespiratory endurance:* The ability to do moderately strenuous activity over a period of time. It reflects
  how well your heart and lungs work to sup-

ply your body with oxygen during exercise.

- *Muscle strength and endurance:* The ability to exert maximum force is muscle strength. Lifting the heaviest weight you can in a single exertion is an example of muscular strength. Muscular endurance is the ability to repeat a movement many times, or to hold a particular position for a prolonged period, for example the work required to lift a weight twenty times or to hold it up for five minutes.

- *Flexibility:* The ability to move a joint through its full range of motion and elasticity of the muscle.

A well-rounded exercise program should develop each fitness component. But some people need more help in one area or another.

BODY COMPOSITION

Body composition refers to your percentage of body fat, not your weight. You can't determine your exact body composition by consulting standard height-and-weight tables, but the tables can give you a rough indication of whether you're overweight.

More precise methods of determining body fat—such as underwater weighing and high-tech techniques using infrared light, sound waves, or electrical currents—require special equipment. But the low-tech, pinch-an-inch test can also help you determine your body composition. Locate a fold of skin and sub-cutaneous fat (the layer of fat beneath the skin) and pinch it between your thumb and forefinger. The back of the upper arm, the side of the lower chest, the back of the calf, and the abdomen are good places to test. After you pinch, measure the thickness of the flesh. If you can pinch more than one inch, your body has exceeded your optimal weight.

AEROBIC FITNESS

If you don't exercise regularly, you have almost certainly lost aerobic power, and you probably know it. Without exercise you steadily lose aerobic conditioning throughout your thirties, forties, and fifties. By age sixty-five the average person's aerobic capacity has dropped by about 40 percent, compared to the relatively fit days of young adulthood. Climbing a flight of stairs or walking through an airport concourse, which once caused little exertion, might now leave you winded and strained.

The term *aerobic* means "using oxygen." During aerobic exercise, your heart and lungs work harder than normal to provide your muscles with the oxygen they demand, and you must breathe heavily and steadily to meet your body's increased need for oxygen. During anaerobic exercise, your heart and lungs cannot meet your body's oxygen demands for longer than a short burst of activity, and you are left gasping and wheezing for breath (even if you're in good shape). Jogging around a track is aerobic exercise; sprinting to catch the bus is anaerobic exercise. No one can do anaerobic exercise for more than a couple of minutes.

To improve your level of aerobic fitness and strengthen your heart and lungs, you need to perform some type of aerobic exercise, such as walking, jogging, bicycling, swimming, cross-country skiing, aerobic dancing, rope skipping. These activities involve the rhythmic, repeated use of the major muscle groups. When done regularly—three times a week for at least twenty to thirty minutes—aerobic activities improve the efficiency of the heart, lungs, and muscles and increase their ability to do work and withstand stress.

Regular aerobic exercise helps lower your pulse rate, both during exercise and at rest. As your heart grows larger and stronger, it pumps more blood with each beat, decreasing blood pressure. One study found that older people who had already suffered a heart attack reduced their risk of a second attack by 20 to 25 percent when they started to exercise. These heart-saving benefits show up after as little as six to ten weeks of regular aerobic exercise.

For maximum benefit you need to work hard enough—but not too hard. Your pulse rate, or the number of heartbeats per minute, is your body's speedometer: It tells you how fast you're going and if you need to speed up or slow things down to exercise in your optimal conditioning zone. Cardiovascular conditioning takes place when your heart beats at 70 to 85 percent of its maximum safe rate. You maximum heart rate is approximately 220 minus your age. (See the table below.) You should take your pulse before starting to exercise, again after exercising for ten or fifteen minutes, and immediately after stopping.

Measure your heart rate at any place where you can feel your pulse. Two easy pulse points are the inside wrist and the carotid artery in the neck. Using a stopwatch, count your pulse for ten seconds, then multiply that number by 6 to get the number of beats per minute. During exercise a pulse that is under your target range indicates that you should speed up or work harder, while one that is higher means that you should slow down. Another simple test: You should be able to talk comfortably during exercise; if you can't carry on a conversation, you're working too hard.

TARGET PULSE RANGES

AGE	MAXIMUM HEART RATE	TARGET RANGE
25	195	137–166
30	190	133–162
35	185	130–157
40	180	126–153
45	175	122–140
50	170	119–145
55	165	115–140
60	160	112–136
65	155	109–132
70	150	105–128
75	145	102–123
80	140	98–119
85	135	95–115
90	130	91–110

If you're new to exercise, start slow. Try ten minutes of light to moderate exercise three times a week and gradually extend your workout time to twenty or thirty minutes, then increase the intensity. If this is too much, start with what feels comfortable to you; the importance is that you begin. While our bodies need a certain duration of exercise for optimal health, you don't need to be a clock-watcher. The length of our workout is important only if you want it to be. Keep track of the time if that helps to motivate you, but don't worry about how many minutes you've exercised if monitoring times makes you weary or makes you feel unsuccessful. Listen to your body, and over time you will develop a workout routine that is both physically challenging and spiritually fulfilling.

If you are over fifty, consider a low-impact activity; as we get older, the shock-absorbing fat pads in the feet thin out and the cushioning disks in the spine dry up, making high-intensity exercise more punishing on the joints. Remember that you can get a good workout using your arms; orchestra conductors tend to live into old age in part because they wave and swing their arms—often strenuously enough to work up a sweat—long enough to complete a concert.

Aim for workouts of moderate intensity, about 70 percent of your maximum heart rate. If you work at the higher end of the exercise benefit zone, you will experience a faster improvement in your athletic ability, but this extra effort won't markedly improve your health and it greatly increases your risk of injury. The death rates from cardiovascular disease, cancer, and diabetes are much lower in moderate exercisers than in nonexercisers. But the rates in heavy exercisers are only slightly lower than those of moderate exercisers. In addition, moderate exercise reduces stress, anxiety, and blood pressure as effectively as strenuous exercise does.

Be sure to warm up for five to ten minutes by doing light calisthenics before your aerobic workout. You might also go through the motions of the main workout at a slower pace as a warm-up.

Also remember to cool down. After your workout, walk slowly for three to five minutes or until your heart rate returns to just ten or fifteen beats above the resting rate. (The less fit you are, the more time you'll need for a cool-down.) Stopping suddenly can cause the blood to pool in the legs, reducing blood pressure and possibly causing fainting or even a heart attack.

If one of your goals is weight loss, exercise is key. Try to work out frequently, slowly, and for a long period of time. Your body doesn't begin to pull from fat reserves until you're at least twenty minutes into your workout, so you should strive to design a regimen that involves five or six workouts a week, each lasting thirty to sixty minutes.

MUSCLE STRENGTH

You will lose strength if you don't perform strength-training exercises. Many people assume that their muscles will atrophy over the years, but this doesn't have to be the case. You can keep your muscles strong and supple by performing strength-building exercises, such as weight lifting and isometric exercises.

Without strength training, you will lose muscle mass and strength: The average American loses ten to twenty percent of muscle strength between the ages of twenty and fifty, and then another 25 to 30 percent between the ages of fifty and seventy. In addition, every decade from age forty on, the average person loses six pounds of muscle; this change in body composition from muscle to fat can change the shape of your body even if it doesn't change your weight on the scales because muscle is denser than fat.

Strength training helps stave off changes in body composition by raising the basal metabolic rate, or the number of calories the body burns at rest. The more muscle you have, the higher your metabolic rate, the more calories you burn, and the easier it is to fight flab. At age twenty, the average woman has 23 percent body fat; the average man, 18 percent. At thirty-five, those fat figures have jumped to 30 percent and 25 percent, respectively. And by age sixty, the average woman is 44 percent fat, and the average man is 38 percent fat. That increase in fat corresponds to a decrease in muscle mass over the years.

To slow this shift from muscle to fat, you must do strength-building exercises, not just aerobic exercise. Studies have shown that people who maintain their aerobic fitness still lose muscle mass—about one pound of muscle every two years after age twenty—if they don't diversify their workouts to include strength training.

In addition to keeping you lean, strength training has these benefits:

- It makes it easier to perform simple tasks such as carrying groceries, opening jars, and climbing stairs.

- It decreases the risk of falls and injury.

- It strengthens the joints.

- It helps build bone mass and fight osteoporosis.

In fact, regular strength training can virtually stop the aging process when it comes to your muscles. For example, one study found that seventy-year-old men who had been strength training since middle age were just as strong, on average, as twenty-eight-year-old men who didn't strength train.

No matter what your age or physical condition, you can benefit from strength training. The more out of shape you are, the greater your proportional gain will be. Frail octogenarians can easily double or triple their strength in just a couple of months. One study found that ninety-year-old nursing home residents increased their muscle strength by up to 180 percent in an eight-week exercise program. High-resistance exercise offers impressive benefits, even at age 101. When done properly, weight training has no great risk of injury or pain.

TRAINING TIPS

Your training weight should be 70 to 80 percent of the maximum weight that you can lift. So if the heaviest weight you can lift in a certain maneuver is twenty-five pounds, your training weight for that exercise would be fifteen to twenty pounds. You should be able to lift that weight eight to twelve times. Once you can lift a weight twenty times, it's time to move up to a heavier weight.

This approach helps build "fast twitch" or "white" muscle fibers, which are responsible for strength. Muscles also contain "slow twitch" or "red" muscle fibers, which help with exercise endurance. To build these muscles, include weight sets that are lighter and perform more repetitions. As you approach fatigue, you will feel a burning sensation in the muscle as lactic acid builds in the muscle tissue. For this approach, do your initial weight set at 70 to 80 percent of your maximum, then mix in a set that is 40 to 60 percent of maximum (or lower). It is natural to feel achy a day or two after working a muscle group in this way. If your muscles feel painful longer than that, talk to a physical trainer or another health professional for advice.

One set of each exercise is almost as effective as multiple sets in building muscle and boosting metabolism. However, to build muscle faster, follow a high-intensity strategy: After finishing the set, reduce the weight by ten pounds and perform as many extra repetitions as you can (usually three or four). This is called a drop set; you can keep lowering the weight with each set until you can lift only a few pounds. One two-month study found that people who followed the high-intensity strategy were able to lift twenty-five pounds more than before, compared to a fifteen-pound improvement among those who followed the one-set approach.

Three workouts per week is the basic rec-ommendation for building muscle. However, once you achieve the desired level of strength, you should be able to maintain that level with two strength-training sessions a week.

To make muscles grow, work to the point of muscle failure, or to the point that you can-not perform another repetition of the exer-cise. Some experts believe the body needs to build up lactic acids inside the muscle cells to stimulate growth. Others believe that heavy weights tear apart the muscle and cause it to form new muscle fibers.

Take it slow and easy. Each repetition of an exercise should take about six seconds—two seconds for the first half of the maneuver and four for the return to the original position.

Use good form. Doing an exercise incor-rectly can cause muscle damage and injury.

Don't hold your breath. Holding your breath can cause a dangerous rise in blood pressure, then a sudden drop when you re-lease your breath, possibly causing lightheadedness or fainting. Inhale, then exhale during the exertion phase of the movement, and inhale during the release.

Be wary of free weights. Start with weight-lifting machines or elastic exercise bands if your strength or balance have declined, since free weights can be dangerous if dropped.

FLEXIBILITY

Flexibility is a critical part of fitness, and one that is often overlooked. Flexibility involves more than being able to touch your toes; it involves maintaining the range of motion in your joints, which can allow you to perform your everyday activities without discomfort. It also makes you less prone to muscle strains, sprains, and tears. The only way to preserve your flexibility is regularly to perform stretching exercises.

Without regular stretching, the average adult's flexibility declines by 5 percent per decade. Over the years, that steady loss in flexibility can make it difficult to stoop over to pick up something dropped on the floor or to look behind you when driving.

As little as ten minutes of stretching every other day can help to prevent stiffness and loss of flexibility. Don't stretch "cold" muscles. Instead, stretch two or three minutes into your warm-up, just after you have broken a sweat. Stretch for two minutes before aerobic activities and ten minutes before abrupt, stop-and-go activities, such as tennis or basketball. You don't need to stretch before strength training, but you should afterward. Regardless of the type of exercise you perform, after your workout stretch two minutes for every ten minutes of your workout time. Stretching helps circulate your energy through your meridians, both before exercise and after.

To build flexibility, bend or flex until you feel tension or slight discomfort—but not pain—and hold each stretch for twenty to sixty seconds. Do not hold your breath, and do not bounce or pulse, which can tear the connective tissue in the joints.

Building strength and increasing flexibility

are not mutually exclusive. This myth has been perpetuated by people who build muscle and fail to work at stretching. Successful dancers and athletes know that they need to stretch before and after they train or perform—and so do you.

GET READY, GET SET, GET MOVING

No matter what your physical condition, it's never too late to start exercising, but don't expect to overcome decades of inactivity in a couple of weeks. It took a long time to get out of shape, and it will take some time to get back in shape, so be patient with yourself. You'll start to feel the physical and emotional benefits of exercise in a few weeks, and your fitness level will continue to improve over the next few months. Studies have shown that a year of regular exercise can return the body to a fitness level of ten years earlier.

Roughly two-thirds of all those who start an exercise program quit within six months. To get into shape, you have to make a commitment to exercise regularly; sporadic exercise

WORK OUT, DRINK UP

You can't rely on your thirst to tell you when to drink during exercise. Instead, you should make a point to drink two eight-ounce glasses of water about two hours before exercise, and another eight ounces every twenty minutes or so during exercise. Then drink an additional cup or two a half hour or so after you finish your cool-down.

This water is necessary for your body to regulate temperature, carry nutrients, remove toxins and waste materials, maintain blood volume, and facilitate chemical reactions in your cells. You lose water throughout the day through urination, defecation, perspiration, and respiration (you release water vapor each time your exhale). When you're working out, you lose even more, depending on how hard you're working, as well as the weather and environment where you're exercising.

If you don't drink enough water, your body will let you know. You should check the color and quantity of your urine. If it's dark and scant, you're not drinking enough and your body is concentrating waste products in a relatively small amount of water. Urine should be pale yellow, and you should urinate at least four times a day.

won't bring the rewards of fitness. Your body will adapt to the physical demands you place on it, and it will do so without injury or discomfort, if you exercise sensibly. If you're not used to lifting anything heavier than a ten-pound bag of groceries, you'll find it difficult to lift a twenty-pound barbell. But if you gradually increase the demands on your body, your muscles will become stronger and your heart and lungs will begin to work more efficiently.

You can challenge and strengthen your muscles in one of three ways: by increasing the intensity of exercise (the amount of weight you lift or the speed you run), the duration of exercise (the length of time you work out), or the frequency of exercise (the number of workouts per week). As a rule of thumb, limit the increase in intensity to no more than 10 percent per week to allow your body to adjust gradually to your fitness program.

You need to space your workouts for maximum benefits. If you perform aerobic exercise fewer than three times a week, you will not achieve adequate aerobic conditioning. However, if you work out five times or more, you run a much higher risk of injury and only a nominal additional increase in fitness. Perform your aerobic exercise every other day, with the strength-training sessions in between.

Once you start exercising, keep at it. Consistency counts. If you miss a few days of exercise, don't feel guilty and throw in the towel (literally). Instead, just get back to it, but don't try to make up for lost time by increasing the intensity of your workout. In fact, if you skip exercise for one week, cut back on the intensity of your workout and gradually build up again. You start to lose aerobic conditioning and strength if you sit it out for as little as one week.

HOW MUCH EXERCISE IS ENOUGH?

You don't have to spend hours in the gym working out to enjoy the benefits of exercise. Recent studies have shown that as little as thirty minutes a day of light physical activity

EXERCISE CAUTION

Before starting an exercise program, check with your doctor if you fit any of the following categories:

- You haven't had a medical checkup in more than two years.

- You're over thirty-five.

- You're more than twenty pounds overweight.

- You have high blood pressure.

- You have high cholesterol.

- You've had a heart attack, rapid heart palpitations, or chest pain after exercise.

- You're taking or have taken heart medication.

- You have angina pectoris, fibrillation or tachycardia, an abnormal electrocardiogram (EKG), a heart murmur, rheumatic heart disease, or other heart problems.

- You smoke.

- You have a blood relative who died of a heart attack before age sixty.

- You have diabetes.

- You have asthma, emphysema, or any other lung condition.

- You get out of breath easily.

- You have arthritis or rheumatism.

- You lead a sedentary lifestyle.

reduces your risk of disease by lowering blood pressure and cholesterol. Yes, that's physical activity, not hard-core exercise. The time you spend strolling the neighborhood, walking the dog, climbing the stairs, and mowing the lawn counts toward your goal. Other studies have shown that you don't even have to do your thirty minutes of activity all at once, as long as you total a half hour of time during the day.

Of course, these studies looked at minimum levels of exercise. To enjoy all the benefits of exercise, you have to work harder and longer. But the point is that with a nominal level of exertion you can enjoy major lifesaving improvements in your overall health.

Regular exercise and physical activity should be your goal. Strive to build time for regular exercise into your daily and weekly routine. Realistically, however, some people are not able (or willing) to make exercise a priority in their lives. For them, making a commitment to an active lifestyle is the best they can do.

As mentioned earlier, you can enjoy many

of the healthful benefits of exercise without spending hours in the gym. In fact, you can reduce your cholesterol and lower your blood pressure by engaging in as little as thirty minutes of activity every day. This "lite" exercise routine doesn't reward you with the same physical benefits as a rigorous workout does, but it is enough to stave off the harmful effects of a sedentary lifestyle.

Here are two sample routines, which can meet the exercise needs of different individuals.

The Maximum Benefit Workout

To attain peak fitness (while still trying to minimize the time spent at the gym or working out), you need to strive to do aerobic training three times a week, strength training three times a week, and stretching for flexibility following every workout.

Monday	30 minutes aerobics
	10 minute cool-down/stretching
Tuesday	30 minutes weight lifting
	10 minute cool-down/stretching
Wednesday	30 minutes aerobics
	10 minute cool-down/stretching
Thursday	30 minutes weight lifting
	10 minute cool-down/stretching
Friday	30 minutes aerobics
	10 minute cool-down/stretching
Saturday	30 minutes weight lifting
	10 minute cool-down/stretching
Sunday	Rest

The Daily Living Workout

Several studies show that simply burning an extra 150 to 200 calories a day (or 1,000 to 1,500 extra calories a week) provides some cardiovascular benefits—and helps you lose weight and build muscle. To burn extra calories, you need to do at least thirty minutes of moderate activity. (See the table below for a rough estimate of how much you burn doing some simple household tasks.)

Create a worksheet for yourself and keep a log of time spent in activity. For example:

Activity:	Mowing the lawn
Time spent:	20 minutes
Calories used:	110 (5.5 calories per minute x 20 minutes)

Activity:	Walking
Time spent:	15 minutes
Calories used:	68 (4.5 calories per minute x 15 minutes)

If you want to follow an active-lifestyle exercise plan, you need to be conscientious about monitoring your activity level, at least in the beginning. Once you get a feel for the activity (and time) required to meet your goals, you can become less rigid about watching the clock.

HOW MANY CALORIES ARE YOU USING?

The following list gives you a general idea of how many calories you burn doing certain daily activities. The estimates are for a 135-pound person. (The more you weigh, the more you burn).

ACTIVITY	CALORIES BURNED PER MINUTE
Brisk walking	4.5
Mopping the floor	4.5
Washing the car	4.5
Weeding	4.5
Gardening (digging)	5
Roughhousing with kids	5
Mowing the lawn	5.5
Shoveling snow	6
Walking (fast)	6.5
Backpacking	7
Jogging	7
Walking upstairs	7
Running fast	13
Running upstairs	15

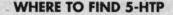

9. WHERE TO FIND 5-HTP

THE GOVERNMENT REGULATIONS SURROUNDING the sale of 5-HTP can be quite confusing. In 1994, Congress loosened the restrictions on selling nutritional supplements when it passed the Dietary Supplement Health and Education Act. Under this law, 5-HTP can be considered a nutritional supplement or a drug, depending on how it is marketed and sold.

If 5-HTP is sold as a nutritional supplement, then it is not subject to control by the U.S. Food and Drug Administration (FDA).

However, if 5-HTP is sold as a sleep aid, antidepressant, or any other product designed to treat a medical condition, then it is classified as a drug and must meet FDA regulations.

When 5-HTP is sold as a nutritional supplement (a food), the FDA does not require that it be evaluated for safety or efficacy. In fact, the FDA will act against the manufacturer of a nutritional supplement only if it receives a number of reports of bad reactions to a product after it has reached the marketplace.

Due to the use of 5-HTP as both a nutritional supplement and a legal drug, it is sold both by prescription and over-the-counter. As a general rule, prescription sources tend to be less expensive than over-the-counter sources.

5-HTP is available at many health food stores, as well as the mail-order sources listed below. Due to the huge variations in cost, you can probably save money by calling a number of local health food stores to compare prices. Be sure to note the number of milligrams of 5-HTP in each capsule and the number of capsules in each bottle so that you can accurately compare product costs.

YOU CAN'T LOOK IT UP

5-HTP is classified by the FDA as an orphan drug. That means that no pharmaceutical house or manufacturer has a patent on the product. Since 5-HTP is an orphan drug, it is not listed in the *Physician's Desk Reference* or other guides to prescription drugs.

WHERE TO GO SHOPPING

The following pharmacies offer 5-HTP by mail or phone. Call the health food stores in your area to find out if 5-HTP is available near you. Because of the growing popularity of 5-HTP, new retail outlets are offering 5-HTP every day.

Super Value Pharmacy
720 N. Industrial
Euless, TX 76039
(817) 283-5308
(817) 283-2821 FAX
E-mail: supval@aol.com
Cost: 100 100-milligram capsules for $52
($5.20/gram)
By prescription

College Pharmacy
833 North Tejon Street
Colorado Springs, CO 80903
(800) 888-9358
(719) 634-4861
Fax: (800) 556-5893
Fax: (719) 634-4513
Cost: 100 100-milligram capsules for $61
($6.10/gram)
By prescription

**Hopewell Pharmacy and Compounding
Center**
1 West Broad Street
Hopewell, NJ 08525
(800) 792-6670
Fax: (800) 417-3864
Cost: 100 100-milligram capsules for $65
($6.50/gram)
By prescription

Medical Center Pharmacy
10721 Main Street
Fairfax, VA 22030
(800) 723-7455
Fax: (703) 591-3604
Cost: 100 100-milligram capsules for $69
($6.90/gram)
By prescription

Vitamin Research Products, Inc.
3579 Highway 50 East
Carson City, NV 89701
(702) 884-1300
(800) 877-2447
Fax: (702) 884-1331
Fax: (800) 877-3292
E-mail: www.vrp.com
Cost: 90 33-milligram capsules for $36.95
($12.32/gram)
No Prescription Required

Pathway, Inc.
5415 Cedar Lane
Bethesda, MD 20814
(301) 530-1112
(800) 869-9160
Cost: 100 100-milligram capsules for $200
($20/gram)
By prescription

Cosmic Sales and Marketing
120 Copeland Road, Suite 234
Atlanta, GA 30342
(800) 359-9896
Fax: (888) 366-8704
E-mail: nubrain@cris.com
Cost: $49 for 180 50-milligram capsules
($5.44/gram)
No prescription required

REFERENCES

Books

Appleton, William S. *Prozac and the New Antidepressants.* New York: Plume, 1997.

Baumel, Syd. *Serotonin: How to Naturally Harness the Power Behind Prozac and Phen/Fen.* New Canaan, CT: Keats Publishing, 1998.

Chaitow, Leon, N.D., D.O. *Thorsons Guide to Amino Acids.* London: Thorsons, 1991.

Epstein, Rachel. *Eating Habits and Disorders.* New York: Chelsea House, 1990.

Erdmann, Robert, Ph.D. *The Amino Revolution: The Breakthrough Program That Will Change the Way You Feel.* New York: Fireside, 1987.

Jonas, Jeffrey M., M.D., and Ron Schaumburg. *Everything You Need to Know About Prozac.* New York: Bantam Books, 1991.

Kramer, Peter D. *Listening to Prozac: A Psychiatrist Explores*

REFERENCES

Antidepressant Drugs and the Remaking of the Self. New York: Viking Press, 1993.

Murry, Michael T., N.D. *Natural Alternatives to Prozac.* New York: William Morrow, 1996.

Overeaters Anonymous. *The Twelve Steps of Overeaters Anonymous.* Los Angeles: Overeaters Anonymous, 1990.

Robertson, J. and T. Monte. *Natural Prozac: Learning to Release Your Body's Own Anti-Depressants.* San Francisco: Harper, 1997.

Wurtman, Judith, Ph.D. *Managing Your Mind and Mood Through Food.* New York: Harper, 1988.

Wurtman, Judith, and Susan Suffes. *The Serotonin Solution.* New York: Fawcett Books, 1997.

Articles

Abraham, H. D. "L-5-hydroxytryptphan for LSD-induced psychosis." *Am J Psychiatry* 140, no. 4 (April 1983): 456–58.

Agren, H., et al. "Low brain uptake of L-(11C)5-hydroxytryptophan in major depression: A positron emission tomography study on patients and healthy volunteers." *Acta Psychiatr Scand* 83 (1991): 449–55.

Alino, J. J., et al. "5-hydroxytryptophan (5-HTP) and a MAOI (nialamide) in the treatment of depressions: A double-blind controlled study." *International Pharmacopsychiatry* 11, no. 1 (1976): 8–15.

Arranz, B., et al. "Serotonergic, noradrenergic, and dopaminergic measures in suicide brains." *Biol Psychiatry* 41, no. 10 (May 15, 1997): 1000–09.

Avery, D., and G. Winokur. "Mortality in depressed patients treated with electroconvulsive therapy and antidepressants." *Arch Gen Psychiatry* 33 (1976): 1029–37.

Badawy, A. A. "Tryptophan metabolism and disposition in relation to alcohol and alcoholism." *Adv Exp Med Biol* 398 (1996): 75–82.

Belongia, E. A., et al. "An investigation of the cause of the eosinophilia-myalgia syndrome associated with tryptophan use." *New England Journal of Medicine* 323 (1990): 357–65.

Benkelfat, C., et al. "Mood-lowering effect of tryptophan de-

REFERENCES

pletion: Enhanced susceptibility in young men at genetic risk for major affective disorders." *Arch. Gen. Psych* 51, no. 9 (September 1994): 687–97.

Birmaher, B., et al. "Neuroendocrine response to 5-hydroxy-L-tryptophan in prepubertal children at high risk of major depressive disorder." *Arch Gen Psychiatry* 54, no. 12 (December 1997): 1113–19.

Blundell, J. "Pharmacological approaches to appetite suppression." *Trends Pharmacol* 12 (1991): 147–57.

Blundell, J. E. "Serotonergic influences on food intake: Effect of 5-hydroxytryptophan on parameter of feeding behavior in deprived and free-feeding rats." *Pharmacol Biocem Behav* 11, no. 4 (October 1979): 431–37.

Blundell, J. E., et al. "Serotonin, eating behavior, and fat intake." *Obes Res* 3, no. 4 (November 1995): 471S–76S.

Blundell, John E. "Serotonin and the biology of feeding." *American Journal of Clinical Nutrition* 55 (1992): 155S–59S.

Broderick, P., and V. Lynch. "Behavioural and biochemical changes induced by lithium and tryptophan." *Neuropharmacology* 21 (1982): 6671.

Bussone, G., et al. "Monoamine oxidase activities in patients with migraine or with cluster headache during the acute phases and after treatment with L-5-hydroxytryptophan." *Riv Patol Nerv Ment* 100, no. 5 (September–October 1979): 269–74.

Buydens-Branchey, L., et al. "Age of alcoholism onset. II. Relationship to susceptibility to serotonin precursor availability." *Arch Gen Psychiatry* 46 (1989): 231–36.

Byerley, W., et al. "5-hydroxytryptophan: A review of its antidepressant efficacy and adverse effects." *J Clin Psychopharmacol* 7 (1987): 127–37.

Cangiano, C., et al. "Eating behavior and adherence to dietary prescriptions in obese adult subjects treated with 5-hydroxytryptophan." *Am J Clin Nutr* 56 (1992): 863–67.

Caruso, I., et al. "Double-blind study of 5-hydroxytryptophan versus placebo in the treatment of primary fibromyalgia syndrome." 18, no. 3 *J Int Med Res* (May–June 1990): 201–09.

Chadwick D., et al. "Manipulation of brain serotonin in the treatment of myoclonus." *Lancet* 2, no. 7932 (September 6, 1975): 434–35.

Chaouloff, F., et al. "Effects of food deprivation on midbrain 5-HT1A autoreceptors in Lewis and SHR rats." *Neuropharmacology* 36, no. 4–5 (April–May 1997): 483–88.

Charney, D. S., et al. "Serotonin function and human anxiety disorders." *Annals of the New York Academy of Sciences* 600 (1990): 558–69.

Chouinard G., et al. "Tryptophan in the treatment of depression and mania." *Advances in Biological Psychiatry* 10 (1983): 47–66.

Comings, David E. "Serotonin: A key to migraine disorders?" *Nutrition Health Review* 70 (summer 1994): 6.

Coppen, A. "Tryptophan and depressive illness." *Psychological Medicine* 8 (1978): 49–57.

Coppen, A., et al. "Levodopa and L-tryptophan therapy in Parkinsonism." *Lancet* 1 (1972): 654–57.

Curzon, G. "Serotonin and appetite." *Annals of the New York Academy of Sciences* 600 (1990): 521–31.

Darmani, N. A., S. L. and Reeves. "The stimulatory and inhibitory components of cocaine's actions on the 5-HTP-induced 5-HT2A receptor response." *Pharmacol Biochem Behav* 55, no. 3 (November 1996): 387–96.

DeBenedittis, G., R. and Massei. "5-HT precursors in migraine prophylaxis: A double-blind cross-over study with L-5-hydroxytryptophan versus placebo." *Clin J Pain* 3 (1986): 123–29.

Delgado, P. D., et al. "Serotonin function and the mechanism of antidepressant action." *Arch Gen Psychiatry* 47 (1990): 411–18.

Delgado, P. L. "Serotonin and the neurobiology of depression: Effects of tryptophan depletion in drug-free depressed patients." *Arch Gen Psych* 51, no. 11 (1994): 865–74.

Den Boer, J. A., and H. G. M. Westenberg. "Behavioral, neuroendocrine, and biochemical effects of 5-

REFERENCES

hydroxytryptophan administration in panic disorder." *Psychiatry Res* 31 (1990): 270–78.

Ellenbogen, M. A., et al. "Mood response to acute tryptophan depletion in healthy volunteers: Sex differences and temporal stability." *Neuropsychopharmaology* 15, no. 5 (November 1996): 465–74.

Fernstrom, John D. "Dietary amino acids and brain function." *Journal of the American Dietetic Association* 94, no. 1 (January 1994): 71–77.

———. "Tryptophan, serotonin and carbohydrate appetite: Will the real carbohydrate craver please stand up!" *Journal of Nutrition* 118 (1988): 1417–19.

Fernstrom, Madelyn H., and John D. Fernstrom. "Brain tryptophan concentrations and serotonin synthesis remain responsive to food consumption after the ingestion of sequential meals." *American Journal of Clinical Nutrition* 61, no. 2 (Febuary 1995): 312–19.

Gibbons, J. L., et al. "Effects of para-chlorophenylalanine and 5-hydroxytryptophan on mouse killing behavior in killer rats." 9, no. 1 *Pharmacol Biochem Behav* (July 1978): 91–98.

Goldbloom, D. S., et al. "The hormonal response to intravenous 5-hydroxytryptophan in bulimia nervosa." *J Psychosom Res* 40, no. 3 (March 1996): 289–97.

Golden, Roberts N., et al. "Serotonin, suicide and aggression: Clinical studies." *Journal of Clinical Psychiatry* 51, 12 suppl. (1991): 61–69.

Goodwin, G. M., et al. "Plasma concentrations of tryptophan and dieting." *British Medical Journal* 300 (1990): 1499–1501.

Haleem, D. J., and S. Haider. "Food restriction decreases serotonin and its synthesis rate in the hypothalamus." *Neuroreport* 7, no. 6 (April 26, 1996): 1153–56.

Hartmann, E. "Effects of L-tryptophan on sleepiness and on sleep." *J Psychiatr Res* 17 (1982–3): 107–13.

Heboticky, N. "Effects of L-trypophan on short term food intake." *Nutritional Research* 5, no. 6 (1985): 595–607.

Helnder, A., et al. "Urinary excretion of 5-hydroxyindole-3-

acetic acid and hydroxytryptophol after oral loading with serotonin." *Life Sciences* 50 (1992): 1207–13.

Hoshino, Y., et al. "Serum serotonin levels of normal subjects in physiological state and stress conditions: From the viewpoint of aging, circadian rhythm, ingestion of diet, physical exercise, sleep deprivation and alcohol ingestion." *Jpn J Psychosom Med* 19 (1979): 283–93.

Iacono, R. P., et al. "Concentrations of indoleamine metabolic intermediates in the ventricular cerebrospinal fluid of advanced Parkinson's patients with severe postural instability and gait disorders." *J Neural Transm* 104, no. 4–5 (1997): 451–59.

Jimerson, D., et al. "Serotonin in human eating disorders." *Annals of the New York Academy of Sciences* 600 (1990): 532–44.

Kahn, R. S., et al. "Effect of a serotonin precursor and uptake inhibitor in anxiety disorders: A double-blind comparison of 5-hydroxytryptophan, clomipramine and placebo." *International Clinical Psychopharmacology* 2, no. 1 (1987): 33–45.

Kahn, R. S., and H. G. M. Westenberg. "L-5-hydroxytryptophan in the treatment of anxiety disorder." *J Affect Disord* 8 (1985): 197–200.

Kaye, Walter H., and Theodore E. Weltzin. "Serotonin activity in anorexia and bulimia nervosa: Relationship to the modulation of feeding and mood." *Journal of Clinical Psychiatry* 51, 12 suppl. (1991): 41–48.

Landry, Mim J. "Serotonin and impulse dyscontrol: Brain chemistry involved in impulse and addictive behavior." *Behavioral Health Management* 14 (1994): 35–38.

Lehmann, J., et al. "Tryptophan malabsorption in dementia: Improvement in certain cases after tryptophan therapy as indicated by mental behaviour and blood analysis." *Acta Psychiatr Scand* 64, no. 2 (August 1981): 123–31.

Lehnert, H., et al. "Increased release of brain serotonin reduces vulnerability to ventricular fibrillation in the cat." *J Cardiovasc Pharmacol* 10 (1987): 389–97.

LeMarquand, D., et al. "Serotonin and alcohol intake, abuse

and dependence: Clinical evidence." *Biological Psychiatry* 36 (1994): 326–37.

Leonard, B. E., "Serotonin receptors and their function in sleep, anxiety disorders and depression." *Psychotherapy and psychosomatics* 65, no. 2 (1996): 66–75.

Leyton, M., et al. "The effect of tryptophan depletion on mood in medication-free, former patients with major affective disorder." *Neuropsychopharmacology* 16, no. 4 (April 1997): 294–97.

Lieberman, H., et al. "Effects of dietary neurotransmitters on human behaviour." *American Journal of Clinical Nutrition* 42, no. 2 (1982) 36–70.

Lieberman, H. R., J. J. Wurtman, and B. Chew. "Changes in mood after carbohydrate consumption among obese individuals." *Am J Clin Nutr* 44 (1986): 772–78.

LiKam Wa, T., et al. "Blood and urine 5-hydroxytryptamine (serotonin) levels after administration of two 5-hydroxytryptphan precursors in normal man." *Bri J Clin Pharmcol* 39 (1995): 327–29.

Linnoila, V., and M. Virkkunen. "Aggression, suicidality, and serotonin." *J Clin Psychiatry* 53 (1992): 46–51.

Lovinger, David M. "Serotonin's role in alcohol's effects on the brain." *Alcohol Health & Research World* 21, no. 2 (Spring 1997): 114–16.

Maes, M., et al. "Effects of subchronic treatment with valproate on L-5-HTP-induced cortisol responses in mania: Evidence for increased central serotonergic neurotransmission." *Psychiatry Res* 71, no. 2 (July 4, 1997): 67–76.

———. "Stimulatory effects of L-5-hydroxytryptophan on postdexamethasone beta-endorphin levels in major depression." *Neuropychopharm* 15 (1996): 340–48.

Magnussen, I., and F. Engback. "The effects of aromatic amino acid decarboxylase inhibitors on plasma concentrations of 5-hydroxytryptophan in man." *Acta Pharmacol Toxicol* (Copenh) 43, no. 1 (July 1978): 36–42.

Mann, J. J., et al. "Lower 3H-paroxetine binding in cerebral cortex of suicide victims is partly due to fewer high affinity, non-transporter sites." *J Neural Transm* 103, no. 11 (1996): 1337–50.

Martin, T. G. "Serotonin syndrome." *Ann Emerg Med* 28, no. 5 (November 1996): 520–26.

Maurizi, C. "The therapeutic potential for tryptophan and melatonin: possible roles in depression, sleep, alzheimer's disease and abnormal aging." *Med Hypoth* 31 (1990): 233–42.

Meltzer, H. Y. "Role of serotonin in depression." *Annals of the New York Academy of Sciences* 600 (1990): 486–500.

Meltzer, H. Y., et al. "Effect of 5-hydroxytryptophan on serum cortisol levels in major affective disorders. I. Enhanced response in depression and mania." *Arch Gen Psychiatry* 41, no. 4 (April 1984): 366–74.

———. "Effect of 5-hydroxytryptophan on serum cortisol levels in major affective disorders. II. Relation to suicide, psychosis, and depressive symptoms." *Arch Gen Psychiatry* 41, no. 4 (April 1984): 379–87.

———. "Effect of 5-hydroxytryptophan on serum cortisol levels in major affective disorders. III. Effect of antidepressants and lithium carbonate." *Arch Gen Psychiatry* 41, no. 4 (April 1984): 391–97.

Menkes, B. B., D. C. Coates, and J. P. Fawcett. "Acute tryptophan depletion aggravates premenstrual syndrome." *Journal of Affective Disorders* 32, no. 1 (1994): 37–44.

Meyer, J. S., et al. "Neurotransmitter precursor amino acids in the treatment of multi-infarct dementia and Alzheimer's disease." *J Am Geriatr Soc* 25, no. 7 (July 1977): 289–98.

Michelson, D., et al. "An eosinophilia-myalgia syndrome related disorder associated with exposure to L-5-hydroxytryptophan." *J Rheumatol* 21, no. 12 (December 1994): 2261–65.

Mills, Kirk. "Serotonin syndrome." *American Family Physician* 52 (1995): 1475–83.

Moller, S., et al. "Tryptophan availability in endogenous depression: Relation to efficacy of L-tryptophan treatment." *Advances of Biological Psychiatry* 10 (1983): 30–46.

Murphy, D., et al. "Obsessive-compulsive disorder as a 5-HT

subsystem-related behavioural disorder." *Bri J Psychiatry* 155 (1989): 15–24.

Nakajima, T., et al. "Clinical evaluation of 5-hydroxy-L-tryptophan as an antidepressant drug." *Folia Psychiatr Neurol Japan* 32, no. 2 (1978): 223–30.

Nardini, M., et al. "Treatment of depression with L-5-hydroxytryprophan combined with chlorimipramine: A double blind study." *Journal of Clinical Pharmacological Research* 3 (1983): 239–50.

Neumeister, A., et al. "Effects of tryptophan depletion in drug-free depressed patients who responded to total sleep deprivation." *Arch Gen Psychiatry* 55, no. 2 (February 1998): 167–72.

———. "Effects of tryptophan depletion on drug-free patients with seasonal affective disorder during a stable response to bright light therapy." *Arch Gen Psychiatry* 54 (1997): 133–38.

———. "Rapid tryptophan depletion in drug-free depressed patients with seasonal affective disorder." *American Journal of Psychiatry* 154, no. 8 (August 1997): 1153–55.

Nicolodi, M., and F. Sicuteri. "Fibromyalgia and migraine, two faces of the same mechanism: Serotonin as the common clue for pathogenesis and therapy." *Adv Exp Med Biol* 398 (1996): 373–79.

Nishizawa, S., et al. "Differences between males and females in rates of serotonin synthesis in human brain." *Proc Natl Acad Sci USA* 94, no. 10 (May 13, 1997): 5308–13.

Pihl, R. O., et al. "Acute effect of altered tryptophan levels and alcohol on aggression in normal human males." *Psychopharmacology* (Berl) 199, no. 4 (June 1995): 353–60.

Pihl, R. O., and J. B. Peterson. "Alcohol, serotonin and aggression. *Alcohol Health & Research World* 17 (1993): 113–17.

Poeldinger, W., et al. "A functional-dimensional approach to depression: Serotonin deficiency as a target syndrome in a comparison of 5-hydroxytryptophan and fluvoxamine." *Psychopathology* 24 (1991): 53–81.

Pranzatelli, M. R., et al. "Human brainstem serotonin recep-

REFERENCES

tors: Characterization and implications for subcortical myoclonus." *Clin Neuropharmacol* 19, no. 6 (December 1996): 507–14.

Puttini, P. S., and I. Caruso. "Primary fibromyalgia syndrome and 5-hydroxy-L-tryptophan: A 90-day open study." Rheumatology Unit, L Sacco Hospital, Milan, Italy. *J Int Med Res* 20, no. 2 (April 1992): 182–89.

Quadbeck, H., et al. "Comparison of the antidepressant action of tryptophan, tryptophan/5-hydroxytryptophan combination and nomifensine." *Neuropsychobiology* 11, no. 2 (1984): 111–15.

Reilly, J. G., et al. "Rapid depletion of plasma tryptophan: A review of studies and experimental methodology." *J Psychopharmacol* (Oxf) 11, no. 4 (1997): 381–92.

Risch, S., and C. Nemeroff. "Neurochemical alterations of serotonergic neuronal systems in depression." *J Clin Psychiatry* 53 (1992): 3–7.

Robiolio, P. A., et al. "Carcinoid heart disease: Correlation of high serotonin levels with vascular abnormalities detected by cardiac catheterization and echocardiography." *Circulation* 92 (1995): 790–95.

Ryan, N. D., et al. "Neuroendocrine response to L-5-hydroxytryptophan challenge in prepupertal major depression." *Arch Gen Psych* 9, no. 11 (1992): 843–51.

Sandyk, R. "L-tryptophan in neuropsychiatric disorder: A review." *International Journal of Neuroscience* 67, no. 1–4 (1992): 127–44.

———. "L-tryptophan in treatment of restless leg syndrome." Letter. *American Journal of Psychiatry* 143, no. 4 (1986): 554–55.

Satel, Sally, et al. "Tryptophan depletion and attenuation of cue-induced craving for cocaine." *American Journal of Psychiatry* 152, no. 5 (May 1995): 778–84.

Seltzer, S. "Alternation of human pain threshold." *Pain* 13, no. 4 (1982): 385–93.

Seltzer, S., et al. "Effects of dietary tryptophan in chronic maxillofacial pain." *Journal of Psychiatric Research* 17 (1982–83): 181–86.

REFERENCES

Sicuteri, F. "5-hydroxytryptamine and pain modulation in man: A clinical pharmacological approach with tryptophan and parachlorophenylalanine." *Acta Vitaminol Enzymol* 29, no. 1–6 (1975): 66–68.

Slutsker, L., et al. "Eosinophilia-myalgia syndrome associated with exposure to tryptophan from a single manufacturer." *Journal of the American Medical Association* 264 (1990): 213–17.

Smith, K. A., C. G. Fairburn, and P. J. Cowen. "Relapse of depression after rapid depletion of tryptophan." *Lancet* 349, no. 9056 (March 29, 1997): 915 (5).

Stanley, M., and B. Stanley. "Postmortem evidence for serotonin's role in suicide." *J Clin Psychiatry* 51, no. 4 (suppl.) (1990): 22–28.

Stein, G., et al. "Relationship between mood disturbances and tryptophan levels in post-partum women." *British Medical Journal* 2 (1976): 457.

Sved, A., et al. "Studies on the antihypertensive action of L-tryptophan." *J of Pharm and Exp Therapeutic* 221 (1982): 329–33.

Takahashi, S. "Reduction of blood platelet serotonin levels in manic and depressed patients." *Folia Psychiatr Neurol Japan* 30, no. 4 (1976): 476–86.

Takahashi, S., H. Kondo, and N. Kato. "Effect of L-5-hydroxytryptophan on brain monoamine metabolism and evaluation of its clinical effect in depressed patients." *J Psychiat Res* 12 (1975): 177–87.

Taylor, D. P. "Serotonin agents in anxiety." *Annals of the New York Academy of Sciences* 600 (1990): 545–57.

Tohgi, H., et al. "Concentrations of serotonin and its related substance in the cerebrospinal fluid of parkinsonian patients and their relations to the severity of symptoms." *Neurosci Lett* 150, no. 1 (February 5, 1993): 71–74.

Titus, F., et al. "5-hydroxytryptophan versus methysergide in the prophylaxis of migraine." Randomized clinical trial. *Euro Neurol* 25 (1986): 327–29.

Ursin, R. "The effect of 5-hydroxytryptophan and l-

REFERENCES

tryptophan on wakefulness and sleep patterns in the cat." *Brain Res* 106 (1976): 106–15.

van Praag, H. "Central monoamine metabolism in depression. I. Serotonin and Related Compounds." *Compreh Psychiatry* 21 (1980): 30–43.

van Praag, H. M. "Affective disorders and aggression disorders: Evidence for a common biological mechanism." *Suicide Life Threat Behav* 16, no. 2 (Summer 1986): 103–32.

———. "Management of depression with serotonin precursors." *Biol Psychiatry* 16, no. 3 (March 1981): 291–310.

———. "Serotonin precursors in the treatment of depression." *Adv Biochem Psychopharmacol* 34 (1982): 259–86.

van Praag, H. M., et al. "5-hydroxytryptophan in combination with clomipramine in 'therapy-resistant' depression." *Psychopharmacology* 38 (1974): 267–69.

van Vliet, I. M., et al. "Behavioral, neuroendocrine and biochemical effects of different doses of 5-HTP in panic disorder." *Eur Neuropsychopharmacol* 6, no. 2 (May 1996): 103–10.

Van Woert, M. H., et al. "Long-term therapy of myoclonus and other neurologic disorders with L-5-hydroxytryptophan and caribidopa." *N Engl J Med* 296, no. 2 (January 13, 1977): 70–75.

———. "Serotonin and myoclonus." *Monogr Neural Sci* 3 (1976): 71–80.

Voltaire-Carlsson, A., et al. "Effects of long-term abstinence on psychological functioning: A prospective longitudinal analysis comparing alcohol-dependent patients and healthy volunteers." 13, no. 5 *Alcohol* (September–October 1996): 415–21.

Wa, T. C., et al. "Blood and urine 5-hydroxytryptophan and 5-hydroxytryptamine levels after administration of two 5-hydroxytryptamine precursors in normal man." *Br J Clin Pharmacol* 39, no. 3 (March 1995): 327–29.

Wallin, M. S., and A. M. Rissanen. "Food and mood: Relationship between food, serotonin and affective disorders." *Acta Psychiatrica Scandinavica* 377 (suppl) (1994): 36–40.

Weiner, W. J., et al. "Dopaminergic antagonism of L-5-

hydroxytryptophan-induced myoclonic jumping behavior." *Neurology* 29, no. 12 (December 1979): 1622–25.

Weltzin, Theodore E., et al. "Acute tryptophan depletion and increased food intake and irritability in bulimia nervosa." *American Journal of Psychiatry* 152, no. 11 (November 1995): 1668–72.

———. "Serotonin and bulimia nervosa." *Nutrition Reviews* 52 (1994): 399–408.

Westberg, G., et al. "Secretory patterns of tryptophan metabolites in midgut carcinoid tumor cells." *Neurochem Res* 22, no. 8 (August 1997): 977–83.

Wurtman, J. "Carbohydrate craving, mood changes and obesity." *J Clin Psychiatry* 49 (1988): 37–39.

Wurtman, J. J., et al. "Carbohydrate craving in obese people: Suppression by treatments affecting serotoninergic transmission." *Int J Eating Disorders* 1 (1981): 2–11.

Wurtman, R. "Behavioural effects of nutrients." *Lancet*, 2 (May 21, 1983): 1145.

Wurtman, R. J., and J. J. Wurtman. "Brain serotonin, carbohydrate-craving, obesity and depression." *Obesity Research* 3 (suppl.) (1995): 477S–480S.

Young, S. N. "Behavioral effects of dietary neurotransmitter precursors: Basic and clinical aspects." *Neurosci Biobehav Rev* 20, no. 2 (summer 1996): 313–23.

———. "Use of tryptophan in combination with other antidepressant treatments: A review." *Journal of Psychiatry and Neuroscience* 16, no. 5 (1991): 241–46.

Young, S. N., et al. "Tryptophan depletion causes a lowering of mood in normal males." *Psychopharm* 87 (1985): 173–77.

Zabik, J. E., et al. "The effects of DL-5-hydroxytryptophan on ethanol consumption by rats." *Res Commun Chem* 20 *Pathol Pharmacol* (1978) 69–78.

Zarcone, V. P., et al. "Effects of 5-hydroxytryptophan on fragmentation of REM sleep in alcoholics." *Am J Psychiatry* 132, no. 1 (January 1975): 74–76.

Zmilacher, K., et al. "L-5-hydroxytryptophan alone and in combination with a peripheral decarboxylase inhibitor in the treatment of depression." *Neuropsychobiology* 20 (1988): 28–35.

ABOUT THE AUTHOR

Winifred Conkling is a freelance writer specializing in health and consumer topics. She is the author of more than ten books on natural medicine and health, including *Natural Healing for Children*, *Natural Remedies for Arthritis*, and *Stopping Time*. Her work has been published in a number of national magazines, including *American Health*, *Consumer Reports*, *McCall's*, and *Reader's Digest*. She lives in northern Virginia with her husband and two children.